X
12.12.07

Kangaroo Babies

Kangaroo Babies

A Different Way of Mothering

by Nathalie Charpak
Preface by Georges Charpak
Translated from the French by Elfrida Powell

SOUVENIR PRESS
LONDON

First published in Great Britain 2006 by Souvenir Press
43 Great Russell St, London WC1B 3PD

First published in France under the title of *Bébés kangourous*
2005 by Odile Jacob
English translation copyright © 2006 Souvenir Press and
Elfreda Powell

The right of Nathalie Charpak to be identified as author of
this work has been asserted by her in accordance with the
Copyright, Designs and Patents Act 1988.

ISBN   028563772X
9780285637726

Typeset by M Rules
Printed and bound by MPG Books Ltd, Bodmin, Cornwall

Contents

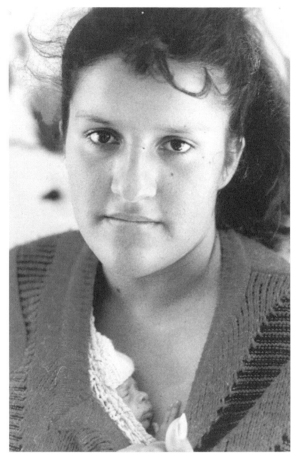

This kangaroo baby, nestled against its young
mother with her tender, anxious gaze, is so tiny that
you might not notice it at all

Preface

Twelve years ago, if anyone had told me that the name of a marsupial with a comical hop would arouse such a strong surge of emotion in me, I would have been amazed. At that time such strong emotions were shared by just a few people – people who helped snuggle tiny premature babies next to their mother's or their father's or sometimes even their grandfather's naked skin. These babies were taken far away from the incubator which they would normally have shared – sometimes for weeks – with other babies from poor suburbs.

Ten years later, in a little house measuring just thirty square metres, attached to a large Colombian hospital in Bogotá, which delivers 18,000 babies a year, you can appreciate the great leap forward that this method has taken. Using a scientific approach that had its origins in a great humanitarian idea, it has been sustained by pioneer doctors and nurses, whose actions radiate a love of children.

In Casita Canguro (Little Kangaroo House), a hundred consultations take place every day; a team of four doctors follow up the kangaroo babies' progress every week and their mothers are taught how to look after their tiny infants. Obviously the progress of these 'kangaroo babies', compared

3

with that of newborn babies left to develop using standard methods of care, will rely a great deal on the new way in which the babies are cared for by their family and by the medical teams.

Happily there are things which can be done without having to have organisations to plan them and it is a miracle that I was involved in such a venture. In 1989, by good fortune I happened to run into Antonino Zichichi, one of my physicist colleagues at CERN (the European Centre for Nuclear Research), who told me that he had received a commission and funding from the Italian government to establish an NGO, the ICSC World Laboratory, to help Third World countries, and that he was looking for original ideas.

I told him that in Bogotá I had just seen an astonishing way of coping with the needs of premature babies and it had moved me deeply. I said that I could not see how it could fit in with the ambitious and revolutionary programmes of irrigation, teaching and scientific research that he was involved in, there was no way round that. But I was wrong. My colleague was sensitive to the humanitarian aspect of an activity that, if it were successful, it would be possible to develop a technology that could be transmitted from one developing country to another. And this has since proved to be the case, while it has also proved of value in several developed countries too. With his characteristic energy, Antonino Zichichi took matters in hand and, over ten years, in a critical period for its development, the Kangaroo Project has, thanks to him, benefited from constant and precious aid from the World Laboratory.

Today more than thirty countries practise the Kangaroo

Preface

Mother Care method or the Kangaroo Mother Method, as it is also known. No gathering of paediatricians takes place without some important discussion being devoted to its progress, and even highly industrialised countries use it. Our initial feelings about the project have been borne out.

The book that you are about to read is a simple, accurate description of the technical rules that govern the kangaroo method and that have been developed over the last ten years by Dr Nathalie Charpak, a paediatrician working in Colombia with the Kangaroo Foundation team, and, among others, her colleague Dr Zita Figueroa. The chapters on Africa and Asia show how this method has been adapted in a variety of countries and civilisations. The artistic photos by Jean-Luc Petit and the more technical ones by Nathalie help the reader follow every aspect of how the kangaroo method works and give us insight into the kangaroo baby and its family's daily life.

I just know that if you are a mother or a father, and if your child has been born preterm, you will appreciate this book. And, equally, if you are a health care professional who, more than once, has hesitated to use kangaroo mother care for want of information, you will also find this book an immense help.

I hope that you will welcome this method and be moved by it, for it brings together a real knowledge of the fragile baby's specific needs and a way of humanising those needs: it is a glance into the future.

Georges Charpak
(*Nobel Prize Laureate in Physics*)
May 2005

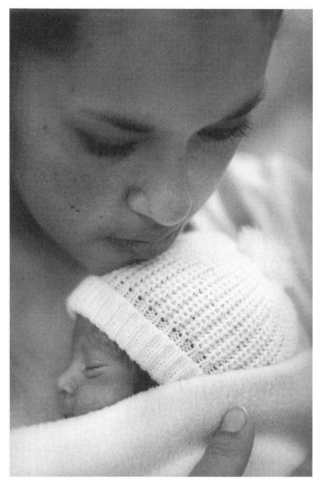

How happy this young mother looks and how content
her tiny baby

Introduction

The Kangaroo Mother Method

*Why It Is Needed, and Who
Benefits from It*

It was in Colombia, in 1978, that the kangaroo mother method was created as a way of alleviating a desperate situation in a big maternity hospital in Bogotá, where there was a hopeless lack of technical support, and within twenty years or so its use has spread like wildfire. At first it was directed specifically towards the needs of babies born prematurely or with a low birth weight, but nowadays it is also used in developed countries to stimulate breastfeeding and develop a good relationship between mother and infant.

In fact, contrary to what is often thought, the kangaroo mother method is valuable for all newborn babies from the moment they come into the world. Because a mother and child ought never to be separated, the idea of nestling a baby, skin to skin, next to its mother from its very first moments of life should gain ground, in our opinion, as standard practice in all maternity hospitals.

Both for mother and for baby the pleasure is instantaneous; the baby immediately seeks out the breast and we know that the sooner the baby can begin to suck efficiently, the more straightforward breastfeeding will be. So the whole process can start smoothly. Of course a newborn baby which is born full term will only tolerate being carried in such close contact for just a few hours a day, whether by the mother or the father, and it will find a way all on its own of protesting when the kangaroo position becomes uncomfortable.

I was already using the kangaroo position in certain very special circumstances, with, for example, adoptive parents who were distraught when their baby would not stop crying, even after it had been fed and had its nappy changed. In these moments of high tension, the kangaroo position enabled them to calm their little baby down and learn to know it physically, in an almost sensual way, and so be able to understand it better. I believe that the kangaroo mother method not only works physiologically, but that it opens a channel of communication between the baby and its parents, a channel which is even more important nowadays when non-communication between human beings seems so often the case. Kangaroo mother care has no limits and can be applied at the earliest possible moment to all tiny babies the world over. Such is my wish, my hope and my purpose in writing this book.

A final word before I embark on my story of the kangaroo method. This book contains photographs that show just what a kangaroo mother (or father) has to do, and I must thank the photographer Jean-Luc Petit for generously donating his royalties to our Kangaroo Foundation, and also Dr Nga Nguyen of the Uong Bi kangaroo programme in Vietnam, Dr Berlith Persson of the Helsingborg kangaroo programme in Sweden, Dr Christiane Huraux of the CHIC de Créteil kangaroo programme in France, Pierre

Introduction

Jaccard (Colombia) and Dr Figueroa (the IMIP Kangaroo programme of Recife, Brazil) who graciously allowed me to use some of their photos. A very big thank you to all of them, and to all the kangaroo babies and parents who agreed to pose for us.

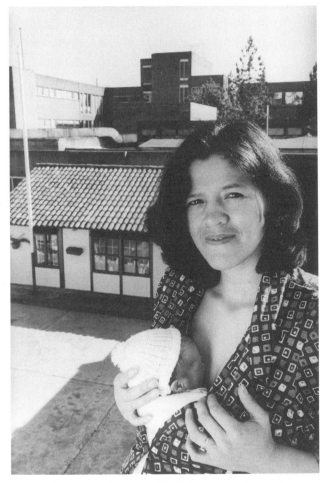

The Casita Canguro (Little Kangaroo House)
at the Clinica del Niño, Bogotá

1

The Kangaroo Babies
of Bogotá

Sebastian is born

Today Maria Isabel is particularly happy for at last she can go home with her little boy, Sebastian, born prematurely fifteen days ago at the San Pedro Claver clinic. She works at a big florist's and everything was going well during her first pregnancy when suddenly she started to bleed and appalling pains shot through her stomach. She was rushed to hospital and had to have a caesarean to save her baby: her placenta had implanted itself too low down, so the young doctor looking after her explained. Sebastian was born at thirty weeks, ten weeks before he was due, and he was immediately hospitalised in San Pedro's intensive care unit, the biggest and best equipped in the Colombian Social Security Institute's clinics in Bogotá. Maria Isabel got up on the very first day – though with some difficulty – to go and see and cuddle her tiny baby: he weighed just 1,250g and she couldn't stop crying when she saw him separated from her in an incubator. The nurse explained to her that Sebastian had adapted very well to his life outside the womb, and she should spend as much time as she could here, in the unit, with him. She also explained to her that as soon as Sebastian could be fed, her breast milk would provide his main nourishment and that with the help of all the caring team she would begin to carry him next to her skin to keep him warm and relieve his stress. Maria Isabel left the unit feeling calmer and from the very next day she began her onerous job as a 'kangaroo mother'.

Adapting mother and baby to the kangaroo method inside the hospital

Maria Isabel really enjoys carrying her baby, particularly since Sebastian began to grow properly once he could take in the milk every day that she had learned to express manually from her swollen breasts. At first she thought that she could never produce milk, but from the moment she started to carry her little baby around, her production increased and she was able to provide the daily quantity that Sebastian needed. This apprenticeship, which is known as the 'intra-hospital kangaroo adaptation', is an absolutely essential stage during which the new mother learns to discover her baby and the tiny premature baby learns to get to know its mother. During these sessions, Maria Isabel has discovered how to stimulate her son's sucking, and a few days ago, he began to suck at her breast. It was such an emotional experience that it made Maria Isabel cry. The little one still gets tired, but his weight gain is steady and the kangaroo paediatrician and nurse agree that if his growth continues to be satisfactory Sebastian can go home with his mother at the end of the week.

The Kangaroo Babies of Bogotá

Today, as every day, Maria Isabel, who in the meantime has returned home to live, comes back to the hospital to carry her baby, express her milk and breastfeed him. One of the kangaroo nurses, Nubia or Flor Angela or it could be Margarita, is always there to help the new kangaroo mothers and often she will ask the more experienced among them to help her out with the others in explaining things – something that has to be done over and over again: they must be told how to carry their baby, how to massage it, skin to skin . . . Maria Isabel enjoys taking part in this collective kangaroo mother life in the maternity unit, for she also benefited from the other women's experience when she was carrying Sebastian early on. She recollects how he fell asleep immediately as soon as he was nestled next to her skin, right from the beginning, as though he recognised her scent, her warmth and the sound of her heart that he had come to know during the seven months that he was in her womb.

Sebastian has now been alive in the outside world for more than fifteen days. He sucks his mother's breast and presents no pathology that requires assistance from the hospital. All he needs is warmth, his mother's milk and constant vigilance, and who better than his mother to provide these three elements? The time for this little baby to leave the hospital is getting closer and closer and Maria Isabel feels deeply emotional. During the adaptation process she learned to massage him, he adores that and stretches and relaxes during the massage. She has also discovered that he reacts to music. Often the kangaroo nurse will play an old battered cassette of classical music during the massage sessions; she tells them that Mozart is the most relaxing . . .

Maria Isabel's husband Nicolas also carries Sebastian around every morning before going to work. He was a little reticent about it at the beginning but, at the medical team's insistence, he finally agreed to carry him and he has gradually come to love doing it. Nothing in the world would make him miss this morning visit. This feeling of being able to protect this tiny, infinitely fragile being snuggled up against his chest, and the fact that every day, thanks to his own body heat, the baby is growing, is extraordinary, and every time he talks about it to those around him, his eyes fill with tears.

Sebastian is ready to leave hospital

Sebastian has been very lucky, for his premature birth has presented no complication. At last he can go home to his parents' house and will only be followed up at the kangaroo outpatients clinic at the Casita Canguro. Maria Isabel and Nicolas have a short interview with Alba, the unit's social worker, who wants to ensure that they are fully aware of the difficulties of caring that await them at home.

Maria Isabel and Nicolas say that they know about these already, that they have bought the cotton Lycra band so that they can carry Sebastian next to their skin and that they have already made an appointment at the Casita Canguro.

It is time to go. Sebastian is dressed in his kangaroo

uniform which consists of a little knitted bonnet, a nappy, socks and a minute sleeveless shirt which opens at the front to allow the greatest possible surface area for skin-to-skin contact. He is placed in the Lycra band in a vertical position, like a little frog, on his father's chest (Maria Isabel is still sore from the wound left by her caesarean), and all that is poking out is his tiny head. Nicolas buttons his shirt and his jacket. To an outside observer, he looks quite funny: like a pregnant man.

Her husband Nicolas is happy to leave (at last) with his son and his wife. The relationship between the three that was interrupted by this premature birth will in some ways be strengthened through having to carry their baby the whole time in the kangaroo way. He knows that they must go to the kangaroo clinic every day, in any case for the whole of this first week, and that a lot of work remains to be done, but his son is now with him, and that is what is most important. So, now they are on their way, first to the Casita, then home.

The outpatient kangaroo programme

Sebastian and his parents make use of the shuttle service between the maternity unit and the Casita, where the outpatient follow-up service takes place. They are going there to meet the team who will keep an eye on them for the first year of Sebastian's life. The Casita is, as always, jam-packed, as no appointment is ever refused. Now . . . the consultation is welcoming, and everyone is seen together;

19

Maria Isabel and Nicolas are frightened and enchanted at the same time. Everything is explained to them a dozen times and they leave with brochures and a 24-hour telephone number they can use if they have any anxieties; their next appointment is made for the following day. When they reach their house, they give a sigh of relief: at last they can begin to lead a more tranquil life with just the three of them and make the most of the new inhabitant who is Sebastian.

The kangaroo mother method: a 100 per cent Colombian invention

In 1978 Dr Edgar Rey Sanabria, a paediatrician and a professor at the National University of Colombia, as well as director of the Neonatal Department at the Mother and Baby Institute (IMI), decided to do something about the growing rate of infant mortality and abandoned babies in his unit. With 30,000 births every year registered in this, the poorest district of Bogotá, it was often necessary to put two or even three babies in each incubator and infections were commonplace. Furthermore, the babies were not growing properly, they remained in hospital for a long time, were often abandoned and often died. Dr Rey had read several studies on the physiology of marsupials and he was convinced that his unit's balance sheet would be much improved if, once it was stabilised, the infant were nestled in warmth and comfort against its mother's bare skin: breast milk could thus be fed directly and the baby could go home, to be well cared for by its own parents. Such were the beginnings of what is today known under the name of the 'kangaroo mother method' or 'kangaroo mother care'. Although it has not been measured scientifically, once the method was in place and applied, the mortality rate and number of abandoned babies fell quickly and dramatically at the IMI.

For fifteen years, this method would continue and develop in a very empirical manner under the leadership of two doctors: Dr Martinez and Dr Navarette. In 1989 a new team, directed by myself, began an evaluation of the method, its systemisation and the creation of precise rules – those that allow Sebastian and his family to go home without taking any risks regarding the baby's survival. Some years later, in 1993, another paediatrician, Dr Zita Figueroa, joined our team and a new kangaroo programme saw the light of day at the Clinica del Niño; then, in 2000, a pilot kangaroo centre at the San Ignacio university hospital was created.

The work is impressive and today more than 10,000 babies have passed through our hands and the World Health Organisation has at last published a practical guide on kangaroo mother care:

When the premature baby and its mother are first separated – a separation which is often necessary and always upsetting – the kangaroo mother method should be considered for the treatment of this initial separation. A bonus of this is that the length of time which is needed to be spent in hospital is reduced, incubators are freed up and can be used for babies that are sick and in the most need, so the scant resources we have at our disposal can be deployed more rationally – something which should be of interest not only to developing countries.

In fact, this usage is not only of interest to Colombia. Thanks to the Kangaroo Foundation, inaugurated in 1994, forty-four teams in more than twenty-five countries have already come to Colombia to learn the method and adapt it to their own cultures.

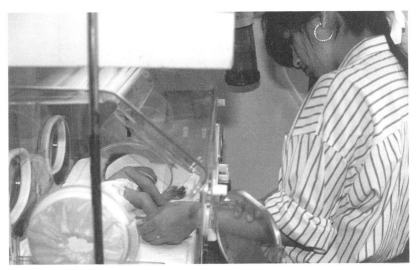

When she visited Sebastian early on, before it was safe to handle
him, Maria Isobel could only stand beside the incubator

It was so upsetting not to be able to do anything other than talk to
him and stroke him in the hope that he would hear and feel that his
mother loved him, that she was with him, and that he must get
better quickly

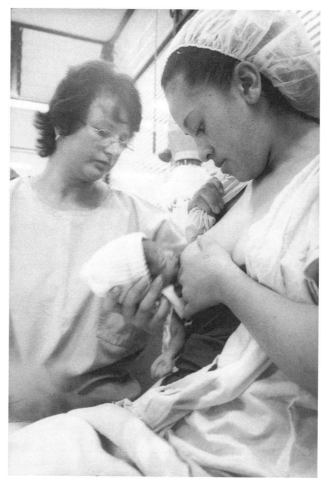

The kangaroo nurse explains to Maria Isabel how
to feed Sebastian and checks her skill at doing it

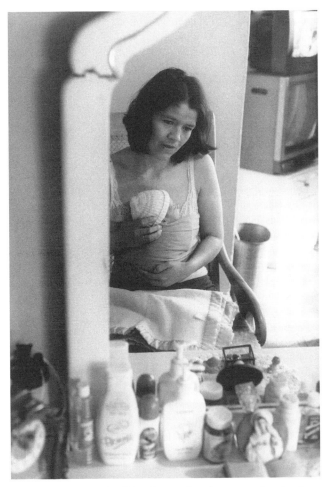

Back at home, the life of a mother kangaroo begins in earnest. In some ways, Maria Isabel almost feels that she is continuing her pregnancy, but now Sebastian is outside her womb

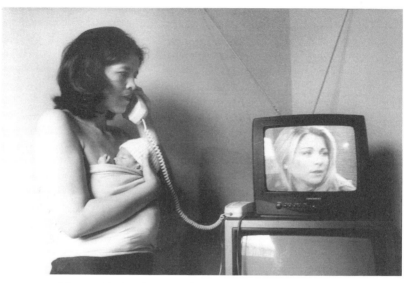

News of Sebastian must be given to all the family . . .

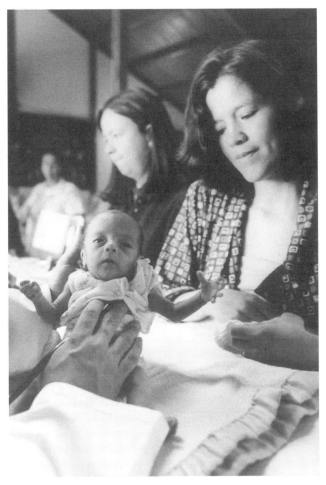

. . . and she must return for the consultation, every
day at the beginning, then, as soon as Sebastian
is growing properly, every week

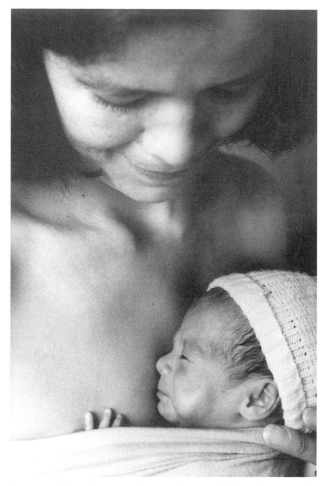

Just one glance is enough to understand that there can be
no intermediary in this union of mother and baby

2

A Different Way of Caring for Premature Babies

The Kangaroo Method

The neonatal divide

We cannot consider the problem of poverty in the world without also taking into account the problem of preterm birth, and in developing countries 90 per cent of babies are born with a low birth weight. At one extreme, we have the richest countries, able to deploy considerable and effective means for the survival of very premature babies who, in earlier times, would undoubtedly have died. At the other extreme, less privileged countries are struggling with situations that cause the death of infants who are less premature: some being born only a few weeks before full term; others are even born at full term, but with a birth weight of less than 2.5 kg. In developing countries, other than premature birth, the cause of low birth weight is in fact malnutrition. This neonatal North-South divide is phenomenal: 90 per cent of the cost of care spent on all these tiny babies worldwide is spent in the developed countries . . .

With this low birth weight, whether or not from being premature, these babies are frail and represent a third of the 5 million children who die in the first month of life every year worldwide. In the South, they constitute a serious public health problem at economic, social, psychological and medical levels. In a number of premature baby units, not only the equipment and human resources are insufficient but they are often poorly organised, or not organised at all. Sophisticated and costly medical technology, when it exists, is rarely available or accessible to everyone, and this shortage increases the risks of mortality, especially in the case of defective incubators and monitors, overloaded services, and frequent nosocomial infections contracted while the patients are in hospital. Parallel with this, in spite of a lack of equipment, medical care suffers from 'dehumanisation' and this corollary of an emphasis on technology is evident, just as in the North. In other words, the care given to the newborn in the countries of the South presents the same problems as in the North, but does not always have the same advantages . . . This aberration, which is specific to developing countries, has forced some paediatricians to find alternatives, such as the kangaroo mother method, conceived by Dr Edgar Rey.

Prolonged skin-to-skin contact, the mother's own milk and an early discharge from hospital form the basic principles of this method, a method that moreover hands over responsibility to the parents by giving them back their role as carers. Since 1978, Dr Rey's pioneering work has been improved upon and developed, and the kangaroo mother method is now used in different forms even in developed countries. In fact this method is not just a solution for poor people. It is often said of the kangaroo position that it is a 'low technology' method, only useful for fighting against hypothermia in developing countries where incubators are scarce. I would like to ask those who hold this reductionist point of view this simple question: is there anything that reveals a higher technology than human skin? Isn't skin permanently supple, firm and warm? Doesn't its temperature automatically regulate itself without the aid of a thermostat? Doesn't the mother's skin have a recognisable scent that is therefore tranquillising? And is it not host to the regular rhythm of its mother's beating heart, that is destressing for the baby? It is decidedly inappropriate to describe carrying the baby next to the skin as 'low technology'. Wouldn't that term be better applied to the incubator, which is a noisy, hostile and echoing enclosure, that is but a pale imitation of the uterus. I also maintain that kangaroo mother care is not only suitable for babies who are stabilised, i.e., who can tolerate being manhandled out of the incubator, without their blood oxygen or their pulse registering a variation. In neonatal care units where there is no equipment at all, the kangaroo mother method becomes a total substitute for the incubator – uniquely by default.

Different ways of applying kangaroo mother care

There are huge disparities in neonatal medicine in the means available between rich and poor countries, but there are also disparities between poor countries. This 'technological divide' explains why kangaroo mother care has been applied in different ways across the world.

In some developing countries they do have incubators,
but in insufficient quantities

Here the kangaroo technique is used as an alternative for routine care for preterm babies and babies with a low birth weight once they have been stabilised. The incubators have to be freed up at the soonest possible moment by the 'stabilised' babies to make way for other babies with more serious conditions. By applying the method in this way the kangaroo technique leads to a more rational use of available technology and human resources, and in addition fosters an earlier relationship between mother and baby. This is the way the method was originally applied in Bogotá. It can easily be replicated in numerous developing countries that have the same type of infrastructure.

The kangaroo technique can also be used in hospitals
where there are no incubators (or where the incubators
are not working)

In this situation, the mother becomes the baby's unique source of warmth and nutrition, even if the baby is sick. Sometimes the team of carers at the hospital insert a feeding tube, but the fact that the baby can survive is down to the permanent kangaroo position nestled against its mother, and thus avoiding hypothermia and hypoglycaemia (a fall in blood sugar).

A Different Way of Caring for Premature Babies

In these destitute countries, 80 per cent of births take place in the villages and hypothermia is the principal cause of death. Kangaroo mother care appears to be the only chance of survival for some of these 'healthy' below-normal or premature babies, by that we mean babies who have no pathology other than having a low birth weight or being immature. But, in these cases, there are several problems that have to be addressed . . .

The total absence of technical help makes it very difficult to identify the very immature, very premature babies. For example, a baby weighing 1,400g could be extremely premature or it could be a baby that has gone to full term but is suffering from severe malnutrition. These two new-born babies will have the same weight, but their prognosis will be different, as will the care necessary for their survival. The very premature baby will probably be incapable of sucking the breast; it will survive hypothermia thanks to the kangaroo mother method, but nothing will prevent it from contracting severe hypoglycaemia, which could damage its brain. Furthermore the premature birth will often have been caused by an infection in the mother, and the baby will develop problems which cannot be looked after in the community.

The kangaroo mother method can be no substitute for the care to which all these premature or malnourished babies should have a right. So it is for this reason that we are seeking to develop kangaroo centres within these countries' great public institutions. These are the big institutions that should ensure the systematic diffusion of kangaroo mother care in their regional hospitals and primary health centres, and eventually in the villages, making sure that they are properly supervised. A *sine qua non* condition is an adequate, targeted training of health professionals. For it is their responsibility to decide whether the little baby should be kept under kangaroo mother care in the village rather than transferring it into a better equipped centre that specialises in the care of delicate babies. It is not an easy decision.

Lastly, the kangaroo technique has an appeal for developed countries

At the outset, this was only conceivable in a hospital environment, once the baby had adapted to life outside the womb and its mother felt ready. The kangaroo mother method is a general step towards humanising neonatalogy: it brings mother and baby closer together, and allows the mother to lavish her attentions on her baby. In this way, stress is reduced both for the anxious mother and for her fragile baby, frequently placed in the fairly unfriendly surroundings of a newborn baby unit. Seen thus, the kangaroo method helps mend the early separation that was necessary during the initial care of the newborn. How many mothers have not felt desperate after a difficult confinement when they have only been able to see their baby full of tubes through the transparent cover of the incubator? They have the sensation of being powerless and this sensation is accentuated by the attitude of the personnel in charge who make them feel that, as far as the baby is concerned, they are being replaced by this personnel for as

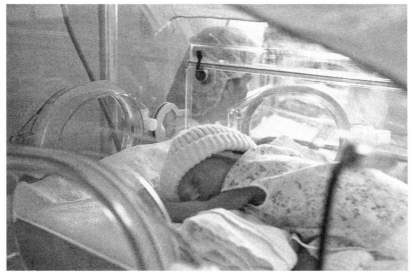

Alone, with the permanent hum of the incubator and intensely bright neon lighting, the newborn baby that has barely emerged from its mother's womb gets to know what suffering and loneliness are long as the baby is in hospital. What distress and guilt these mothers experience then!

Every baby is fragile

As we enter a new millennium it is a good time to stand back and evaluate what has gone on in the past. In the West, there has been an exponential explosion of different technologies. In the course of the last hundred years, the role of a doctor faced with the challenge of a sick baby's survival has changed from being an impotent witness to a foreground performer who possesses the necessary knowledge to understand and successfully modify a newborn baby's immature and impaired physiology. Somewhere along the way, health professionals, in the name of science and technology, and in the so-called interest of the baby, have separated off the parents, physically and emotionally. Babies have been progressively isolated in a strange, even hostile environment.

In affluent countries, the frail or sick newborn baby seems to have been condemned to a strange destiny, for, to ensure the best chances of its survival, it is isolated in a medically high-tech, inhuman environment, and separated from its parents. Painful procedures like injections or blood tests are carried out routinely, without taking into account the nightmarish character that these acts possess for a tiny defenceless creature. Regulation of temperature, the prevention of infections, the monitoring of vital functions or maintaining physiological functions result in placing the baby in an environment which is noisy, painfully brightly lit and aggressive.

How the newborn can suffer

Our current knowledge of the brain's development clearly shows that a newborn baby resents pain just like you and me. Contrary to what we used to think, the pain threshold appears to be even lower among premature babies. By the twenty-fourth week after conception, the sensory receptors are perfectly developed; worse still, the premature baby will experience even slight pain in a less localised, longer and more vivid way than an older baby.

A baby cannot verbalise its suffering; it expresses it either in a change of behaviour or in a severe modification of certain physiological parameters such as heart rate or oxygenation – yes, the heart can stop beating and a baby can suffocate as a result of an intense pain. While on this subject, some extremely interesting studies have been published that indicate that skin-to-skin contact with the mother has the effect of diminishing the sensation of intense stress associated with pain. This is the reason why the kangaroo position, skin to skin, with the baby nestled against his mother's breasts and lulled by her heartbeat, in a gentle warmth and a familiar scent is, during the last few years, becoming a more and more frequent practice in intensive care units for the newborn; more and more often mothers are encouraged to carry their baby and cuddle it to lessen its stress and pain. The kangaroo position provides the baby with a feeling of security, which will help it recover more quickly after painful but necessary handling, such as having a blood sample taken; the heart rate, which rises when the baby has pain, drops to normal more rapidly if the baby is in the kangaroo position than if it is alone in its incubator.

Nowadays in the West the major problem in the units where they are caring for the newborn is the absence of space (in the literal sense as well as in the figurative one) left for the parents. The development of the kangaroo mother method, if it is followed up, will mean great structural changes, but it is the humanisation of high-tech care which is at stake, and it is high time that it was attended to.

Also the kangaroo mother method allows for a closer relationship between the parents and their baby, be it sick or simply frail, and this means that they do not feel so guilty about the premature birth: it reassures them that they are giving their baby all the attention they can and this makes them less anxious about their baby's future. Parents learn progressively to recognise and interpret the signals that their premature baby gives: they become responsible and more devoted to this completely dependent little baby right from the beginning. Recent work shows that later on they will provide a more suitable and more stimulating home for their baby and will also be capable of helping it throughout its development. Finally, it would seem that there is less maltreatment among parents who have been allowed to participate in caring for their fragile baby right from the start.

The neural-sensory development of a premature baby

Light

In an incubator the level of bright light to which a premature baby is subjected is five to ten times higher than the level recommended for office workers. The shock that that represents for a newborn baby can be seen even more clearly when we know that only about 2 per cent of light from outside passes into the uterine cavity and that this is regulated by the rhythm of the mother's life (when she is asleep it is totally dark in the womb), with day/night alternation. Under a phototherapy lamp, it is even worse: the increased brightness can reach 250 to 2,000 times the average mean reference that is acceptable for an adult. The question of potential effects of this over-stimulation is inevitably asked, in particular regarding the appearance of retinal problems that are specific to babies born preterm, or the poor organisation of the baby's sleep. Other questions raised are to do with the impact of live light on their social behaviour, given that every premature baby tries to close its eyes to avoid light and visual contacts during its stay in the unit. However, simple and accessible measures can be taken in all newborn baby units to mimic the alternation of day and night, and protect a baby against intense light. How many mothers have told us of their premature baby's difficulty in falling into a regular pattern of refreshing sleep once it is at home, particularly if it has had a long stay in hospital.

41

Noise

The noise to which a baby is exposed in an incubator is far greater than the noise permissible for working adults. To this must be added isolated, stressful sounds like monitor alarms, bangs when something is put down on the top of the incubator, radios which are often turned on even at night, and which form a background noise to the work of the team in the unit, added to which there can be particularly piercing voices. This noisy atmosphere, which is loud enough to disturb an adult's sleep, seems to have an impact on the baby, causing agitation and crying, which may in turn have a bearing on the reduction of blood oxygen and the increase of intracranial pressure. Not to mention possible deleterious effects on its auditory perception in the future . . .

Touch and scent

From the moment of birth, all tiny babies perceive smells and sense caresses. A piece of fabric impregnated with the scent of their mother and a gentle massage every day are basic things that make a baby grow and therefore recuperate more quickly. It seems so simple . . .

The early mother-baby relationship and the impact of initial separation

In 1972 the conclusions reached by Marshall H. Klaus and John Kennell aroused a great debate about the mother–baby relationship. These two paediatricians wrote that the toll of maltreated infants was significantly higher in families where newborn babies had been hospitalised for long periods and that this maltreatment could be a result of separating mother and baby from the moment of its birth. Klaus and Kennell based their proof on the fact that immediately after the birth there appears to be a period of sensitisation, which lasts from several minutes to several hours, where the relationship can develop harmoniously. In cases where the newborn baby was hospitalised this period of sensitisation was not respected.

To develop their thesis, Klaus and Kennell had recourse to works of ethology and to practical observations on newborn babies who had been hospitalised for long periods in intensive care. In certain animals, such as rats, the mother's behaviour can be upset by an initial separation, making her even go so far as to reject the baby. In humans, they wrote, in the same way mothers separated from their newborn are rather fearful and clumsy in the care they offer their baby: some of them said that they saw their baby as a stranger, not 'belonging' to them and that in cases of long separation, said that they even momentarily forgot that they had a baby. With a firm belief in these observations and the conclusions of their studies on attachment, Klaus and Kennell put forward a theory, that there existed a precise moment after birth during which this mother-baby relationship developed. This period was unique for each mother-baby couple and its impact was fundamental on their future relationship. This relationship could be made easier through skin-to-skin contact and through the exchange of looks when the baby was first put to the breast after delivery.

Since 1972 the initial skin-to-skin contact and putting the baby on the breast immediately have been accepted readily enough and introduced in a good number of maternity hospitals. However, we still as yet have no real proof that there is a fixed period immediately after birth when this mother-infant bond is created. Moreover, in 1984 Kennell and Klaus themselves refined their position and said that immediate contact after delivery was not the only factor determining the child's ultimate development and that a mother could modify her behaviour in the months following the birth without there being any notable consequences for the baby. With this skew, guidelines regarding possible behaviours and interactions became more varied; at the same time it was admitted that the skills required to care for a baby could be learned.

As a result of this refinement, Klaus and Kennell have rallied their more sceptical colleagues. They are agreed on the idea that attachment between mother and baby is an interactive process, nurtured by presence and exchanges, and inclined to disturbance if its normal development is upset. Moreover, everyone admits the negative impact of early separation.

The kangaroo mother method – to return to our subject – can play a considerable complementary role in the creation of this particular bond between a mother and her baby. It has been observed that, compared with groups of women who have not practised this method, mothers who carry their baby in the kangaroo position benefit at least in the short-term in the quality of their maternal perceptiveness and behaviour vis à vis their baby. This effect is probably due to the intimate skin-to-skin contact between the baby and the person carrying it. Since the different results we have had of the studies carried out in Canada and Colombia, numerous neonatal care units have recognised the contribution that the kangaroo position makes on affective and emotional levels and have added direct skin-to-skin contact to their other routine care. They have seen it as a way of humanising their care, improving communication and promoting the bond between mother and baby.

In a general way, in all the countries of the world, whether developed or developing, kangaroo mother care can be considered an indispensable preparatory step for a fragile baby prior to being discharged from hospital and going home to its family, but it is also seen as a 'curative treatment' that can compensate for the effects induced by the initial separation of mother and baby. In fact, through it parents learn to look after their baby, at the same time becoming more sensitive to its needs. And the baby is stimulated by the more skilful care it is given, and can be guaranteed a better quality of survival and better development as a result of this education and of empowering the parents' sense of responsibility.

Urgent action that needs to be taken

Saving what is best in both worlds – North and South – is a matter of urgency. All newborn babies, regardless of their place of birth, have a right to profit from the best possible quality of care, not only on a biomedical and technical level, but also on psychological, human and affective levels. In numerous new attempts in numerous countries, health professionals and scientists of different disciplines have called strongly for more humanisation of the care given to babies and their families. Other programmes similar to kangaroo mother care, like Human Neonatal Care or NIDCAP (Newborn Individualized Developmental Care and Assessment Program) are working towards humanising neonatalogy. NIDCAP, for example, developed by Dr Heidelise Als, interprets alterations in behaviour (agitation, sleep) and the variations of physiological parameters (heart rate, oxygenation) as the newborn baby's 'language' and recommends that the care given to babies in neonatal care units is organised around this language. In particular, skin-to-skin contact, or the kangaroo position, could be suggested at any moment and for every time a fragile baby is handled in a way that risks stressing it.

These alternative solutions would allow newborn babies to benefit from more human care, better adapted to their affective needs and physiologically appropriate. I must stress this fundamental point: the different programmes that I have just mentioned, and, most important of all, kangaroo mother care, are not working *against* technology, nor are they replacing it, except in situations of extreme urgency. These are allied, complementary tools, whose use and spread are underwritten by health professionals who are competent and well trained, and who recognise the immense value of high-tech units for the survival and quality of life of all newborn babies, whatever their social origin and their country of birth, but who nonetheless recognise that technological rigour must act in tandem with the humanisation of care.

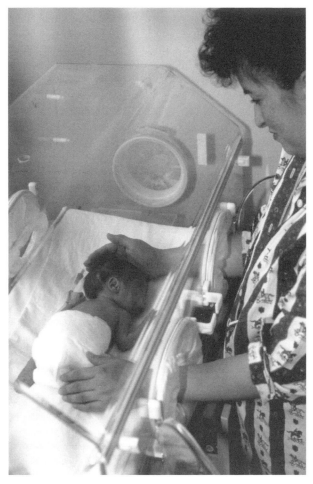

For the first time, a mother timidly touches her baby
who has been separated from her since birth.
Getting acquainted will be a long journey
that has barely begun

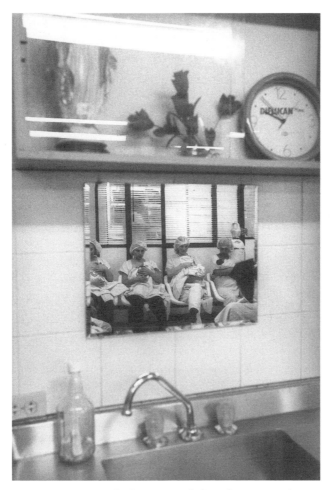

Every morning the kangaroo dads and mums gather
in a windowed room in the middle of the neonatal
care unit and learn to rediscover their little
kangaroo babies

3

Becoming a Kangaroo Mother

Principles and Practice

Mother kangaroo care is natural and makes economic sense. It involves keeping the low birth-weight, almost naked baby cuddled against an adult's chest. This description makes it sound simple, almost too simple . . . Yet it is an authentic neonatal technique of which the basic principle is to replace the incubator as rapidly as possible with a human source of heat and sustenance. Just like marsupials, kangaroo mothers use their own metabolism to help their baby grow or finish its maturation.

The first contact

The right moment to begin kangaroo mother care varies. If the baby is 'healthy', with no critical pathology, starting very early after birth with direct skin-to-skin contact and putting the baby to the breast immediately are preferable. This is ideal for the mother and for the baby, and will guarantee successful breastfeeding. The direct skin-to-skin contact stabilises the baby more quickly. A warm skin, a recognisable voice – its mother's – help the baby relax and oxygenate better, all in non-stressful surroundings. Before placing the newborn baby against its mother's skin, its own skin must be properly dried, especially the head, with a soft warm towel if possible.

On the other hand, when the birth is very premature or coupled with growth retardation, the threat of serious medical complications demands specialised supervision. The baby then remains in hospital and is placed in an incubator for varying periods. Kangaroo mother care cannot be a substitute for this vital medical care. However, no matter what medical treatment and attention are given, the baby needs to hear its mother's voice. And the sooner the better. It also needs to feel its mother's hands touching and cuddling it at the soonest possible moment and as often as possible. In this way she will make the baby aware of her presence and at the same time begin to get to know it and help it fight for its survival.

Once the baby is stable enough to be handled without danger, if it can be placed directly against its mother's skin, it will benefit marvellously from its mother's presence. This beneficial contact must be made as soon as possible and for as long as possible, depending on the state of the baby's health. In some hospital services, in Sweden for example, very immature babies, of less than twenty-eight weeks, on tubes and ventilators, are put in direct skin-to-skin contact with no alteration to their physiological balance. The criteria that the tiny baby must fulfil for this first skin-to- skin contact have to be precisely defined within each neonatal care unit.

Adapting the mother and her newborn baby to the kangaroo method

Once the baby's state is less fragile, kangaroo training continues, whether beside the incubator, or in a neonatal ward where several mothers can sit together.

The aim of these training sessions in the kangaroo method is to prepare mother and baby by getting them sufficiently well acquainted to be able to go home as soon as possible. The future kangaroo mother learns how to place and carry her baby in the kangaroo position, to express her milk manually and to feed her little baby correctly with a cup, a syringe or the breast, in the correct position. In this way she develops confidence in her ability to take charge of her infant.

This training is done under the supervision of nurses who specialise in the kangaroo mother method and are capable of evaluating when the criteria are met that will allow the baby to leave hospital. This is not easy and sometimes it needs a lot of sessions before the very premature baby can obtain adequate nourishment from its mother. Collective training also means that more experienced mothers can share their expertise with newcomers who are often very anxious and clumsy. In fact it encourages sharing and exchange of their common difficulties (feeding, carrying, etc.) among all these women. I want to make a special mention of the fact that in some cultures women are more timid than in others, and for this reason the fathers are not always authorised to participate in these adaptation sessions.

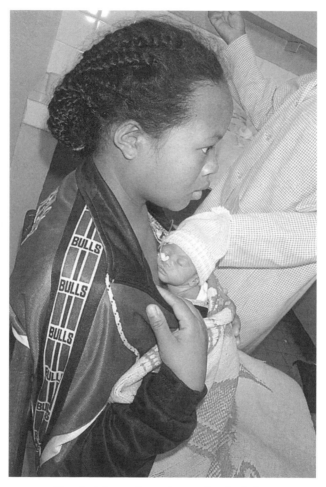

It only takes a few minutes for the baby
to fall into a deep sleep

Becoming a Kangaroo Mother

When the mother is tired, the baby is put back into its incubator. Recent studies have shown that physiologically it is better to carry out these kangaroo method sessions for at least two hours at a time to respect the premature baby's cycle of sleep and digestion. Obviously, where there is no incubator available to alternate with the kangaroo position, the situation is not up for discussion: the baby *must* stay permanently against its mother's skin. Certainly, if it is very ill, this is not an ideal situation, either for the baby or for the mother, but it is perhaps the baby's only chance of survival. In every case, whatever method is applied, it is certain that the early interaction between the tiny baby and its mother produces a better supply of breast milk, vital nourishment for the baby's survival and this is the same in every country in the world.

The ideal position

The baby must be placed strictly upright against its mother's or father's chest. Particular attention must be paid to keeping the airways free. So it is better if the baby is held firmly. Using a band that is tied firmly around the carrier and baby's torsoes helps to maintain this position and allows the mother or father to relax, even to sleep deeply with the baby in the kangaroo position. This bandage is elasticated and is made of cotton Lycra.

In this position the premature baby's head is outside the Lycra band and a draught around its tiny cranium could lower its temperature. Its head should therefore be

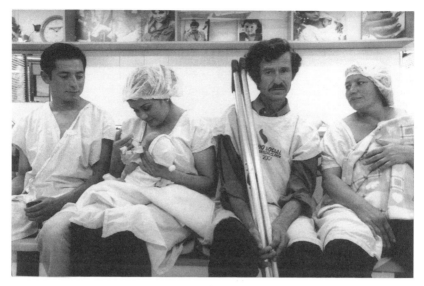

Communal training means that doubts and difficulties can be shared

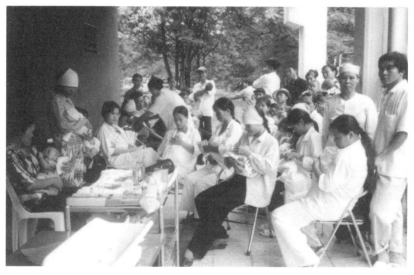

In every country, communal adaptation sessions are much
appreciated by the mothers, for they give them an opportunity to
ask their questions before leaving hospital with the baby. An added
bonus is that the more experienced mothers can explain to the new
ones the sort of difficulties that they are going to encounter.
Depending on the culture, fathers are sometimes allowed in the
same room, or sometimes in an adjoining one

covered with a small bonnet – in wool or cotton – depending on the climate. Little mittens and socks are generally added to this kangaroo clothing. Often the nurses have to fight against the mother's – understandable –wish to clothe their baby with garments that they have prepared for it, which are generally too big and unsuitable for the kangaroo position.

Sometimes in hot and humid countries the mother will burst into a sweat which makes her feel very ill at ease. An airy place is therefore necessary. A thin piece of cotton cloth placed around her neck and down her chest as far as the baby's cheek will make her more comfortable without interfering with skin-to-skin contact. The mother's well-being must be constantly uppermost. Neonatal care units must invest in good chairs and the hospitalisation beds for mother and baby must provide a comfortable semi-seated position so that the mother can sleep with her baby in the kangaroo position. Large pillows will help if all clse fails . . . Metallic upright bars will cut into the back and are particularly disagreeable when a mother is carrying her baby for twenty-four hours a day. An important point to bear in mind is that the kangaroo carrying method is not advisable – it is even dangerous – if the skin is not clean or intact, and if the mother has a high temperature. In these special cases, the bearer must be someone else: all human skin has a temperature of 37 degrees C.

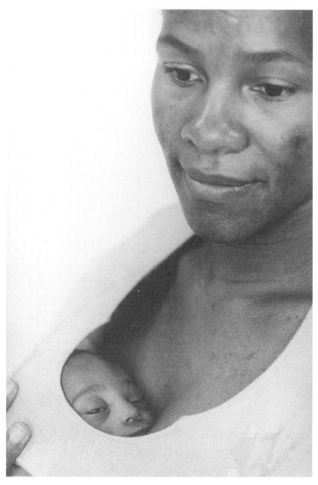

This tiny baby really looks as though it is in its nest

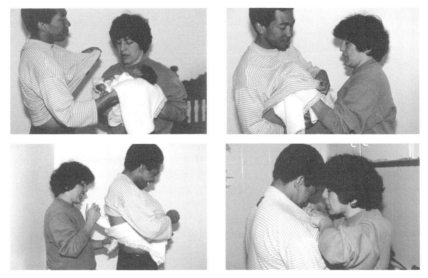

Putting the kangaroo baby in position needs a bit of help,
but only at first

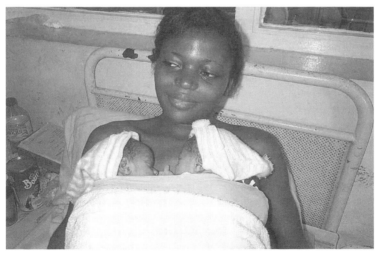

My goodness, when there are two of them, it's still
possible to manage

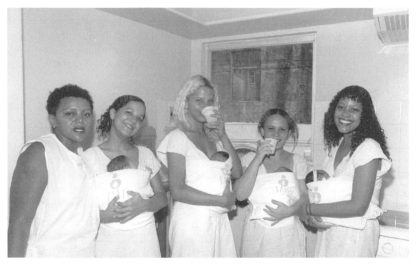

Some can still look sexy even with the baby in the kangaroo position

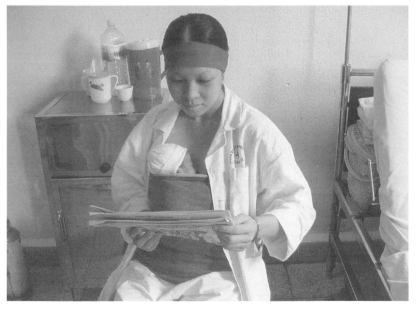

Once the baby is in position, you must have patience

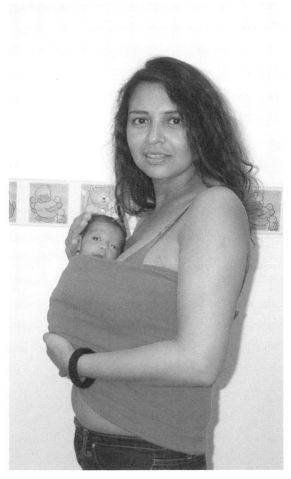

The support is made of synthetic or cotton Lycra,
but a traditional shawl can also be used

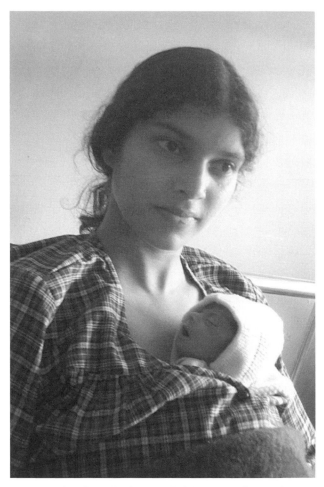

It is only when the baby is fed by its mother and its
temperature kept constant in the kangaroo position that
it can go home. Whatever country or climate, its little
woollen or cotton bonnet has a very important role to
play in avoiding episodes of hypothermia

The father's participation

Fathers should be encouraged to participate. Generally they take a delight in discovering the pleasure of carrying their baby against their skin over the course of the several weeks that were missing in their wife's shortened pregnancy. In this way they share with her the often tiring attention that must be devoted to their fragile baby. They may perhaps never have considered the exhaustion a mother experiences. At home, the kangaroo method engenders a certain respect for all the work a mother has to do in caring for her newborn, work perceived as entirely a woman's responsibility in most cultures.

One of our big surprises when we embarked on our first mother kangaroo programme was the fathers' excellent attendance at the consultations. Colombia is a macho country where the man is rarely involved in baby care, but we had decided, right from the beginning, to get fathers involved. Not only did they behave perfectly, but we observed some strange reactions. One such case was the father of a baby weighing only 1,090 g, whose mother had been hospitalised. He looked after the baby on his own, night and day, for ten days (he was a night guard on some business premises). When the mother came out of hospital, he told us that he wanted to keep the baby and separate from his wife. It took us a lot of patience and help from a team of psychologists to convince him that his wife had equal rights and that his little baby boy needed his mother's milk, which he could not give him. On another occasion a father, a great hairy fellow with a moustache,

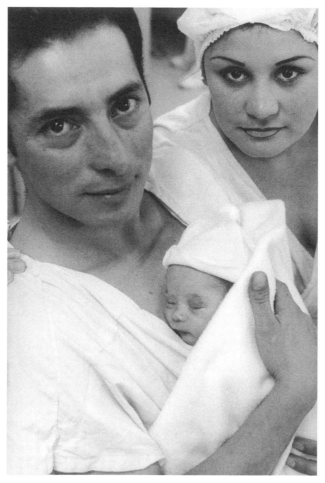

There is always an element of anxiety in handling
such a fragile little creature . . .

started to shave himself twice a day in order to carry his little daughter who weighed 1,300 g. In vain did we repeat to him that it was not necessary, he told us that he knew that she would prefer a smooth skin.

As a general rule, 60 per cent of fathers attend the first consultations. They come to make sure that their baby is growing in the warmth produced by their skin-to-skin contact and they are proud of it. Interestingly too, 80 per cent of the calls on the emergency beeper are from the fathers. When they come home from work, they take their turn to carry their baby in the kangaroo position and have all sorts of questions to ask. During the year, it is not unknown to see these same fathers bringing their little baby to the consultation all on their own without their wife.

Kangaroo nutrition

The kangaroo baby's nutrition relies principally on breast milk. In all the countries of the world, a mother's breast milk, because of its quality, is perfectly suited to the immature organism of a baby born preterm. After all, all industrial milk preparations aim to imitate the composition of natural breast milk as closely as possible. Milks sold commercially are a substitute for the mother's breast milk when it is not available and they are perfect for this.

Feeding the tiny premature baby is not simple. Its mother's milk is first fed directly into its stomach through a tube, then it is gradually given by suction once the baby has

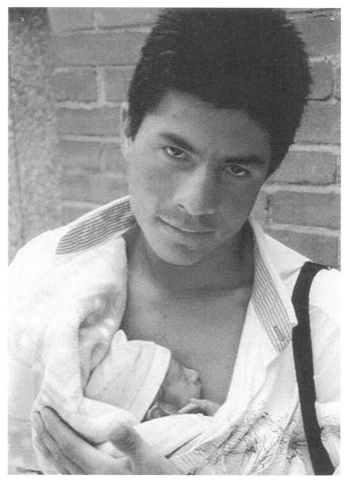

This adolescent father, aged seventeen, has carried his baby of 1,400g for more than a month, its mother is in intensive care and he did not want to confide his son to anyone else

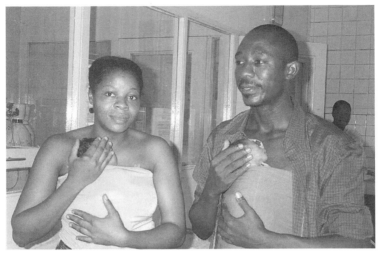

When there are two, the father's participation is even more important to ensure that the babies are being carried correctly in the kangaroo position and to lighten the mother's work

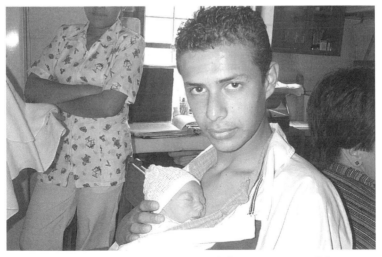

One thing is certain: kangaroo fathers are responsible fathers whatever their age

attained sufficient maturity to suck its mother's breast efficiently without losing weight. As soon as possible, the sucking is stimulated with little exercises that the mother can practise herself. In some countries, a small cup or syringe is used to feed the mother's milk to the baby. Whatever the utensil, the important thing is to avoid using teats, because the teat develops a sucking technique which is different from that used on the nipple. In a word, once the baby has got used to a teat, it is not going to be able to stimulate the production of milk adequately when being breastfed: lactation risks being inadequate and the mother will be obliged to use artificial milk. And as we have said already, mother's milk is the best, and if she wants to breastfeed, she is probably going to feel that she is to blame for her lack of milk. Even when a baby is born at full term, it is not so easy as all that to achieve successful breastfeeding. So, breastfeeding a premature baby has its problems . . .

A mother must not feel alone in the embarrassment she feels. The medical team has a duty to be there when she has her doubts and hesitations. Too often, when breastfeeding fails it is the carers' responsibility. While the mother is full of good intent, she does not always receive all the help she needs.

There are different methods to stimulate a baby's sucking, and help is available for expressing the mother's milk whether manually or using mechanical or electrical gadgets. All these methods demand an intense collaboration between nurses, doctors, psychologists and mothers. The kangaroo mother method is not only the paediatrician's and mother's concern. It is a technique that demands a multidisciplinary

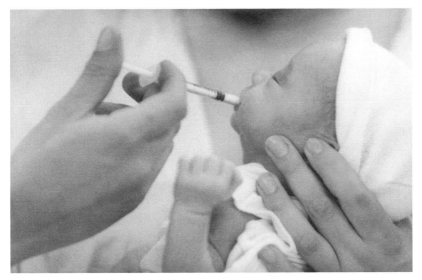

Whether it is at the breast, with a small cup or with a syringe,
feeding the kangaroo baby is not simple

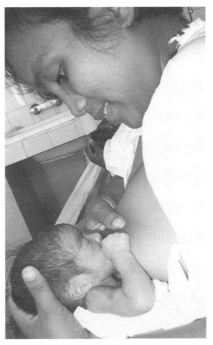

Breast size is unimportant; on the other hand,
time and patience are needed to feed such a tiny baby

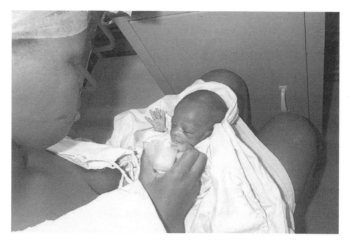

When baby is tired, feeding must be done in shifts, with a cup for example, but not with a teat, for a baby must not get used to a bottle and reject the breast. Pay attention: a few bottles could be enough to threaten the success of breastfeeding which the mother wants to do

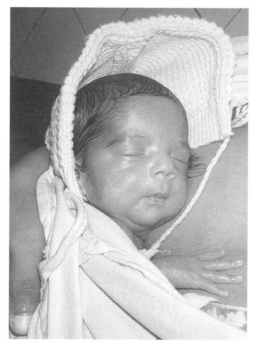

Sated, lulled by its mother's heart beat, warmed by her skin, this little baby appears relaxed and happy, wouldn't you agree?

collaboration between carers and teamwork between parents and carers. The aim of everyone is one thing: the wellbeing and health of the fragile premature baby.

Ending the kangaroo position

What is marvellous about the kangaroo position is that it is never necessary to remove the baby from it. It is the baby itself who knows when it is no longer useful: when it is capable of regulating its own temperature, it begins to sweat and to protest in an effort to disengage itself from this position which prevents it from moving about and stretching its limbs. In countries where there is a hot climate, the baby will logically demand an end of the kangaroo position earlier than in a cold climate. Let it do it. It is as though it is asking to be born . . .

The general rule is to leave the baby all the time that it needs in the kangaroo position. Most often, let us not forget, there are external factors which have forced it out of the womb preterm. It is therefore best to let it complete this lost time in complete tranquillity. If it leaves the kangaroo position when it is too tiny, it risks hypothermia. If it is a little too big, but not sufficiently developed, it is going to use up too many calories to keep warm and its growth will be inferior to what it would have been, had it remained in the kangaroo position. Certainly its maturation in the kangaroo position demands a lot of work from its parents, but it is only during a very limited period, barely a few weeks, that this active participation is requested. Driven by love and a desire to participate, most parents prove to be the best allies of the kangaroo mother method: they know that their efforts will improve the quality of their baby's survival.

When the baby's state of health has improved, it is then transferred into the least complicated of wards, then, if it is possible, sent home under its parents' supervision. In some countries, but not in all, once the mother has been trained to carry her baby and feed it, she can continue her role as kangaroo mother in her own home, while returning regularly for consultations. The condition *sine qua non* for a kangaroo baby to be able to leave hospital is that it has grown at the correct rate during its hospitalisation. Precision electronic scales are in fact the only costly equipment necessary for the kangaroo programme. After that, the kangaroo position is maintained at home, in a permanent way, the baby having constant need of warmth in order to grow adequately.

Mother makes the best carer

'Kangaroo-sceptics' believe that the mother's presence in a neonatal care unit increases the frequency of infections. In reality the opposite is true. Fatal infections are often due to germs which are present in the hospital milieu but never in family homes. What is more, when the carer asks the mothers to cut their nails and wash their hands before touching their baby, this they do with much rigour and never forget to repeat this procedure every time they come into contact with their baby; they are guided by the love for their baby, which is a very precious feeling.

And also, as there is often a great staff shortage in most of the developing countries, the mother is an appreciable help. She can feed her baby more frequently than a nurse in charge of an overwhelming number of children. Since tiny stomachs need to be filled more often with small quantities, this is a task that can be taken over perfectly by a trained mother.

Should kangaroo mother and baby leave the hospital early or remain in hospital?

In some countries, like Colombia, the baby goes home as soon as the mother feels capable of continuing to carry and feed her baby using the kangaroo method. It leaves the hospital independently of its weight or its gestational age, once its mother has been trained and judged fit to look after it in her home.

Does that mean that the kangaroo mother programme with its early discharge of the baby in its kangaroo position can only function with Colombian mothers? No, the training of professionals who have come from other countries has demonstrated that it is completely possible to adapt the kangaroo method to local cultures. What is most difficult is generally to put across the importance of keeping the baby for twenty-four hours out of twenty-four in skin-to-skin contact, at home. The resistance is amazing, when one considers that no one would be astonished at keeping a baby in an incubator night and day until such time as the baby can regulate its own temperature. The Lycra band helps the mother or the father to carry the child, and allows them to feel more confidence and not to be afraid of dropping their baby when they are asleep. The daily follow-up at the beginning, when mother and baby have been discharged from hospital early is also judged to be demanding and costly by kangaroo-sceptics; I would say to them that, before this, the families came to visit their babies every day in the care unit and that seemed normal to them.

On the other hand, when there is no transport, when the mother lives too far away or has no help in the house, it seems wiser to suggest that she stay in hospital. This kangaroo mother-baby service is often communal in developing countries but the rooms can be individual; ideally, there should be a common room for the parents with comfortable seats where they can meet, discuss their baby and share their fears and their hopes, not only among themselves but with professionals who have different specialisations: psychologists, physiotherapists, nutritionists, social workers . . . It is often rare in developing countries to have at hand mothers with time to listen and learn; one needs to take advantage of this and teach them, for the several days or several weeks that they spend in the hospital, everything that concerns the future of their baby: when to vaccinate their child, what to do when the baby has diarrhoea or a fever, what special toys there are for the development of their baby, how to make them cheaply, what exercises are suitable for their baby, what the traditions and beliefs that should not be performed are and

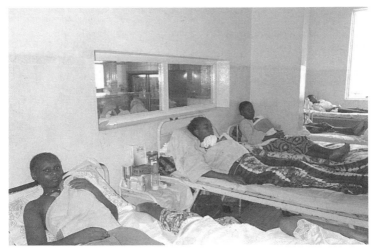

Because of the lack of transport in Africa and in Asia, kangaroo mothers and babies often have to remain in hospital

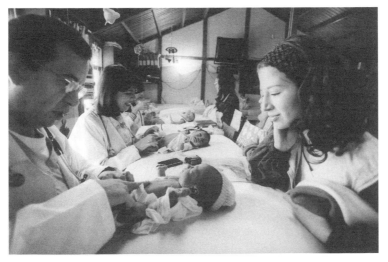

The outpatient clinic is welcoming; this is a time when parents can ask questions and share their anxieties with the carers. It is also the ideal moment to teach everyone the care that needs to be given to a baby during its first year of life

why, how and when to introduce complementary food, what notions of family planning are often welcomed.

As you can see, the kangaroo mother method is also educational work for the mothers; it has an impact not only on the future of the kangaroo baby, but also on the future of all the other children already present at home or who will arrive in the future.

Outpatient clinics

If mother and baby have returned home early with the baby still in the kangaroo position, it is absolutely imperative that they come back to the clinic. At the beginning, they will come daily until the baby has grown by at least 15 grams per kilogram per day. This is the speed of growth that the baby would have enjoyed in its mother's womb had it not been obliged to leave sooner. If early discharge is not possible, this very intensive follow-up period takes place while the kangaroo mother and baby are in hospital.

After this, check-ups become weekly until the baby reaches full term, i.e., the date on which it should have been born. This date is discussed with the family at their first appointment. Ideally, the outpatient clinic should be situated in a place which is separate from the neonatal care unit to avoid the risk of infections that may breed in the hospital. In Colombia, as we have seen, it takes place in a little kangaroo house known as the Casita.

The outpatient part of the kangaroo follow-up is particularly tricky, because when the kangaroo mother and baby return home they are no longer supported by the hospital structure. I always think that the kangaroo method of care until the baby reaches its presumed full term is some ways similar to neonatal home care.

Few blood tests are necessary: if the baby is growing in a regular way, it probably has no anaemia or problems with a lack of calcium or with glycaemia. However, certain vitamins are vital (vitamins A,D, E and K) because, normally, a natural reserve would have been built up during the final term of pregnancy. If there is no reserve, the premature baby may develop serious problems. These risks can be prevented through taking a regular dose of vitamins until the presumed full term. This part of the kangaroo baby's follow-up can be likened to a period of struggle for survival. The physical and neurological state of the baby on its presumed date of birth will give us an insight into the quality of the work that has been done.

In many developing countries, the follow-up stops too early. There appear to be two reasons for this: one is that the mother can see her child putting on weight and looking well and no longer wants to make the effort to go to the clinic; or, secondly – and more often the case – there is no clinic . . . Very often doctors are overwhelmed with work and parents live a long way away. However, this follow-up after full term should go on for as long as possible, at least until school age. The quality of survival of the premature baby is at stake here.

A follow-up like this, when it is extended, will ensure that eventual problems will be detected from the moment they appear – these problems could be visual, auditory and neurological ones or there might even be psychomotor difficulties. An early intervention can prevent such problems, which would be more difficult to treat later on. It is vital to insist on the follow-up of these high-risk children for at least a year.

The ideal situation is to have tiny babies along with older children attending the same clinic; that way their mothers can exchange experiences. Even if professional kangaroo teams are competent, kangaroo mothers and fathers are even more so, for they have lived this experience and are astonishingly happy to be able to talk about things to other parents who are just embarking on their adventure. This is why our clinic mixes the small kangaroo babies with older babies up to the age of one.

The kangaroo mother method is not so complicated as all that. A certain number of rules must be established in order to ensure that the method is adopted successfully, but it is also possible to modify them, such as when to begin the method and what babies are suitable, and at what particular time. There are other issues that can vary such as the criteria for judging when a preterm baby is stable enough for skin-to-skin contact; activities that should be developed during the kangaroo adaptation; the criteria that should be adopted for mother and baby's return home and how frequently the follow-up consultations should be. Before beginning the kangaroo mother method, it's important to make a prudent decision as to what rules to apply, and then modify them later, depending on the baby's progress and how well the method is accepted by the parents and carers.

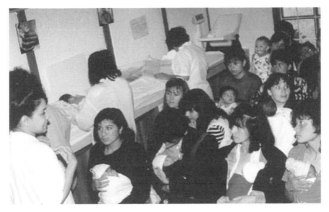

The atmosphere of the clinic is animated and friendly

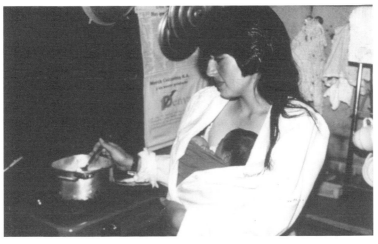

With twins cooking is no simple matter . . .

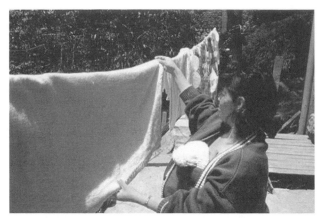

And nor is hanging out the washing

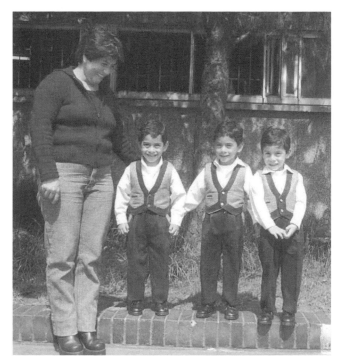

Mothers love going to the clinic to show how big and strong
their kangaroo babies have become. Especially when
they happen to be triplets . . .

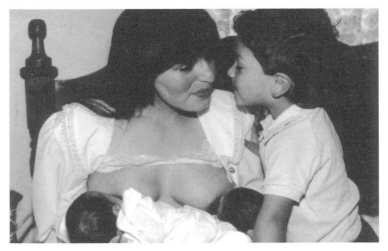

Life back at home is not always simple, but it helps integrate the
baby into its family of brothers and sisters

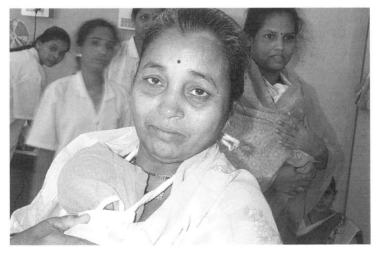

Grandparents can play an important role, especially in the case of
multiple births or when the mother is all alone with her baby

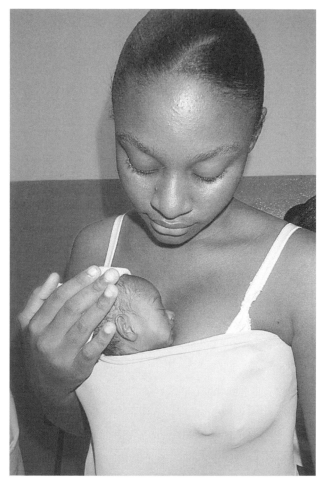

Nestling between his mother's breasts as she tenderly
watches over him, this tiny baby is gathering strength

4

The Benefits of the Kangaroo Method

Are There Risks for the Baby?

In 1989 when the Kangaroo Foundation research team began to evaluate kangaroo mother care, it was not a big thing. The method was considered seductive but very folklorish by most paediatricians in the world. Their viewpoint was not really surprising as there was a lack of rigour in describing the method, which had no written protocol either: 'follow-up' simply meant keeping an eye on them, and the tiny premature babies had no clinical history when they began their programme. It was therefore impossible to know if the babies who did not return for the consultations were dead or if, perhaps, their mother had simply not been successful in getting the money together to take the bus to the hospital. Evaluating the kangaroo mother method and proving its efficacy for mothers and babies worldwide have required an immense amount of work to put things in order.

As early as 1978, however, several paediatricians – notably Susan Ludington-Hoe (USA), Andrew Whitelaw (UK), Viviane Whalberg (Sweden), Richard de Leew (the Netherlands) – had discovered the programme in Colombia and were struck by how happy these mothers were carrying their little baby, so tranquil and warm against their chest. They took home with them the principle – of carrying the baby in skin-to-skin contact, which is essential in the kangaroo mother method – and reported on it; they were also insistent with the international community that this programme be evaluated scientifically. The reports available from this period were inspired, in fact, from studies which compared a series of cases in a controlled population during a period when the kangaroo mother method did not exist . . . Some more rigorous studies were done, but they were incomplete; some of them relied too heavily on too small a number of patients, others only evaluated a minute part of the kangaroo mother method – skin-to-skin contact being limited to a few hours or just to when the premature baby was being breastfed.

So it was only in 1989 that everything began properly, when our research team, funded by the World Laboratory, a little known Swiss NGO, that had been seduced by the kangaroo method, threw itself into a methodical evaluation of the kangaroo mother programme in its native institution. In this way it was established that the mortality rate was not higher in the kangaroo group, but some doubts were expressed on the kangaroo babies' quality of growth after a year of follow-up, the impression being that they were smaller than babies who had remained in the incubator. It is obviously very difficult to know if this difference was related to the kangaroo mother method or to the fact that the two groups under comparison were not from the same socio-economic class. The evaluation needed further research.

Parallel to our work, which was ongoing, in 1991, an

The Benefits of the Kangaroo Method

American scientist, Dr Gene Anderson published an exhaustive review of all the articles on the kangaroo mother method that she had been able to collect, either from reviews or directly from health professionals working on the subject. The studies are classified according to their quality and their scientific value; this work has since been republished in 1999, but without anything notably new.

Demonstrations in the plural

The results of this critical revision deal essentially with the effects on the hospitalised baby, in developed countries, of skin-to-skin contact, one of the most studied components of the kangaroo mother method. Many advantages of direct skin-to-skin contact between mother and baby are highlighted:

1. The regulation of temperature in the kangaroo method is as good as that obtained inside an incubator. Some studies even claim that by using the kangaroo method the regulation is better.
2. Breathing rhythm is more regular in the kangaroo position than in the incubator groups (with less incidence of apnoea).
3. The level of oxygenation in the blood does not decrease when the baby is placed in the kangaroo position.
4. The baby's performance improves and stabilises in the kangaroo position (the baby is more often awake, cries less, etc.)

5. The kangaroo position induces no extra risk of infection.
6. The kangaroo method encourages breastfeeding (it lasts longer).

But Anderson also drew conclusions about the parents and the carers. First of all, kangaroo mothers felt more self-confident (they had a heightened feeling of fulfilment and competence and showed less anxiety . . .) and as a consequence they also had confidence in their ability to breastfeed their baby. Anderson also observed a notable decrease in the initial neonatal hospitalisation time which was directly linked to the skin-to-skin contact and emphasised the positive change of attitude in the health personnel working with the kangaroo mother method: the introduction of this method humanised the behaviour of the team in charge of caring for the baby and modified their attitude towards the families. The relationship became that of a closely knit group uniquely preoccupied with the wellbeing of the newborn, everybody working together in mutual respect. The parents became the key players at the very heart of the service. The kangaroo mother method gave them confidence in themselves, reassured them, made them feel competent and gave them the tools to become the best carers for their fragile baby.

But kangaroo mother care is a lot more than skin-to-skin contact . . .

It has to be said that these studies compiled by Anderson, though favourable, do not form a complete and satisfactory picture of the benefits of the kangaroo mother method in its entirety. In fact, they are not complete since they only relate to skin-to-skin contact. For some time, then, the kangaroo mother method has continued to be controversial, even in Colombia.

Aware of the potential of this method for countries with limited access to technology, and mindful of the need to have a clear response on the efficacy and safety of the kangaroo mother method, in 1993 our team began fresh, much more rigorous research, and this funded by the same NGO that had been at our side for more than ten years. The study was carried out using 746 babies chosen at random and placed either in a kangaroo group, or in a control group looked after in an incubator: they were followed up till they reached the age of twelve months.,

The results confirmed the low mortality rate using the kangaroo mother method; they even suggest that it is less than the control group's when the father's education is poor. Do fathers become more sensitive to the needs of their tiny babies when they have shared these early intimate moments of skin-to-skin contact with their baby? This is an exciting trail that could be better explored.

Also, the results on growth show that not only kangaroo babies grow as much as those in the control group, but that their head is bigger at the end of the first year. I am talking of cerebral growth here, of course. Does this mean that they will be more intelligent later? The question is open . . .

Thanks to the kangaroo mother method, there is less of an overload on neonatal care units and hospital infections are decreasing. At the risk of repeating myself I must stress that when you ask a mother to wash her hands carefully before touching her baby, you can be certain that she will never forget to do so: so, when it comes to the issue of infection, she cannot be considered a risk factor. Finally, the use of the kangaroo method not only humanises the care given to the newborn, it also stimulates the mother's breastfeeding.

This study, carried out in Colombia, showed the reliability of the kangaroo mother method for the first time in a rigorous and scientific manner. Since then, other studies have been done in developing countries; they have shown also that the kangaroo method contributes towards compensating for the lack of technical means to care for newborn babies that have a low birth weight in developing countries. Some work even attests to an impressive decrease in the mortality rate of babies weighing less than 2 kg. On the other hand, few data are as yet available on the long term follow-up and the future of the newborn who have benefited from the kangaroo mother method.

Kangaroo mother care as an integral method of care for the mother and baby

The different studies show that, in the absence of all technology, the kangaroo position and kangaroo feeding, used simultaneously, form a significant solution for hospitals. In such a context, nevertheless, there resides a major problem, and that is that after the early discharge from hospital, outpatient follow-up can be hampered by a lack of transport and extreme poverty. Generally, the outpatient aspect of the kangaroo mother method remains the trickiest issue, in spite of the plethora of benefits that the hospital and the parents will get. This follow-up of the baby at high risk has not yet become routine in developing countries where all too often only the survival of the preterm baby is researched and not the quality of that survival.

A global view of the baby is therefore even more necessary, for that alone would enable us to detect and correct eventual anomalies in the baby's neural-psychomotor or sensory development before the irreparable consequences appear, such as retinopathy of prematurity, refraction problems, cerebral palsy and reduced hearing ability. Our aim is to try to give back to the family a baby in the nearest state possible to a newborn baby that has gone full term, with all the necessary 'tools' for it to grow in the most correct way possible.

What happens if the baby dies at home?

This is one of the most frequently asked questions by all those who are familiar with the kangaroo mother method. Let's be honest, whether this happens at hospital or at home, there is quite a risk of sudden death, and this risk is a cause of anguish for everyone. We also know from experience that the mourning process that any mother goes through when her baby dies is less difficult when the death takes place at home in the kangaroo position and when the mother has been able to do something for her baby than when the baby dies in an incubator and she has been unable to do anything. The process of grieving can be got through in an infinitely better way among kangaroo mothers.

What about infection in the home?

Another question that is often asked is about possible infections that the baby might contract in the house. Obviously mothers should have as little contact as possible with sick people, and we ask everyone to take care, but as I have already said an infection caught at home is never as virulent and dangerous as an infection caught in the hospital.

An evaluation of the costs of the kangaroo mother method in developing countries has been made in numerous studies as well as an evaluation of the acceptance of the method by mothers and hospital staff. The results are positive and attest to a decrease of the costs for babies under this method as well as a good reception of the method by hospital staff and mothers.

To sum up, we can say with certainty that the kangaroo mother method, taken globally and in every aspect – kangaroo position, kangaroo feeding, early discharge from hospital and follow-up of the baby in outpatients – allows for a more rational use of equipment; it can, however, be applied and spread only after appropriate training, particularly in matters relating to early discharge from hospital and follow-ups in outpatient consultations. Convinced by the results of these different scientific studies on the subject, in 2003 the World Health Organisation published a practical guide to the rules of the kangaroo method for hospitals in developing countries, see (www.who.int/reproductive-hepdf).

The mother-baby relationship

An evaluation of the mother-baby relationship, carried out in parallel with studies on other aspects, shows that kangaroo mother care teaches parents how to be more competent when they are looking after their baby, thus ensuring its optimum development. The kangaroo mother method can even act positively on the neurological development of the premature baby as it passes through a very sensitive period of its life: the results suggest, in effect, that when kangaroo mother care is introduced very early in intensive care units, the method protects babies at high risk against mental retardation during the first year of their life.

Kangaroo Babies

Once the baby has pulled through, thanks to the technology, the brain of a tiny preterm baby still has to develop for several months. The idea behind the kangaroo mother method is to reproduce a cocoon, a nest, the nearest possible thing to the milieu in which it floated when it was in its mother's womb. What could be more natural than placing the baby against its mother's warm skin in a tranquil, familiar and relaxing atmosphere and leaving it to recuperate? Its immature brain will surely develop better in this way? This is at least how some think, and the small centimetre of the cranium's perimeter that our kangaroo babies have gained at the time of their follow-up testifies to this.

Every day, new studies relating to the kangaroo mother method are published, particularly in developed countries; they have a bearing on certain points of fundamental research that are implicated in the kangaroo mother method, such as thermal stability in skin-to-skin contact, frequency of apnoea, digestion and hormonal production, sleep quality . . . And while I know that these researches carry positive results in their evaluation of kangaroo mother care, I am equally convinced that the kangaroo mother method forms an integral method of caring for the premature baby and that it has even more important effects when it is applied in full. These new studies open an enthralling field of research into human physiology at the very beginning of life, but as to the validity of the kangaroo mother method's diffusion and application, a sufficient number of scientific tests already exist to prove its reliability and appropriateness when it is a question of available resources and humanising neonatal care. And of equal importance is that it gives parents the feeling that they are the most competent and the most responsible in coping with their fragile baby and getting it through the worst.

Kangaroo mother care's current standing

The kangaroo mother method is gaining ground strongly in developing countries and we should rejoice about it, but we must also point out that there are certain risks of mis-interpretation. First, the kangaroo mother method should not be an excuse not to fight for and not to attempt to adopt the necessary technology to care for fragile babies who are preterm or have a low birth weight: the kangaroo mother method cannot replace neonatalogy; all it can do is complete it. Now, today, bearing in mind the lower cost of discharging a mother and baby from hospital early, there is a tendency to send them home too soon from some hospitals, without any follow-up being possible, for the simple reason that no follow-up consultation has been anticipated or put in train. It is false to assume that kangaroo mother care costs nothing, though its cost is on the whole less than hospital costs. In other words, and I must stress this point, you should refuse to practise the kangaroo method if there is no infrastructure to train mothers or follow up these fragile babies. Furthermore, it is simple common sense to acknowledge that not all mother-baby couples are suited to the kangaroo method. So, if the team of carers reckons that a mother will not come back for check-ups, it is not prudent to allow her to take her little one home. In the same way, if a mother is depressed, you should not force her, or make her feel guilty, but leave her the necessary time to want to use the kangaroo method. Finally, when a mother is alone at home without any help, you must carefully weigh the risks that an early discharge would represent and, if possible, organise a network of solidarity around this woman and make the other members of her family sensitive to her needs.

5

Happier Babies and Parents in Europe

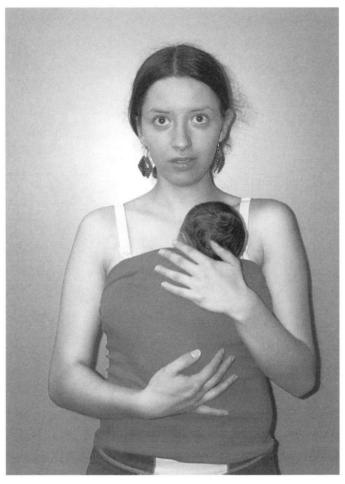

A kangaroo mother always feels responsible
for her tiny baby

'If I were ever to have a premature baby . . . I would stay with it, naked in bed, for months if I had to'. That was how I used to think, and yet, before I gave birth to Josephine, I had never heard of the kangaroo method. It was instinct talking; if the baby was born too soon, there would be no question of leaving it on its own, absolutely none . . . Yet, although I was firmly prepared to stick to my beliefs, when I came face to face with the reality of the medical world it was something of a rough ride . . . Even so, I was lucky that we had a two-hour session of the kangaroo method every day . . .

The experience of this French mother who had given birth to a preterm baby is far from being unique. (http://users.skynet.be/couveuse/ kangaroo.htm).

When you ask a mother to tell you how she lived through the initial separation from her newborn baby, whatever the medical grounds and regardless of how much time has passed since – two or twenty years – she will always be vibrant with emotion as she tells you, and she will be overwhelmed by memories that are still fresh in her mind and will probably remain so until she dies. The conclusion to be drawn is clear and simple: we make our mothers suffer and we also make these tiny babies suffer when they are scarcely born. The medical team, doctors or nurses, are not deliberately aware of this suffering; putting a baby for two days under a phototherapy lamp to cure its jaundice can seem necessary and hardly traumatic, and we sometimes fail to imagine the feelings of a mother when this separation is announced to her. At the same time we never imagine this mother saying 'No' to us; we have the future of her baby in our hands and we feel all-powerful.

In medicine, changes in practice are generally difficult to carry out and have a bad reception from medical staff. There is a mixture of ignorance and fear at the prospect of additional work, for changing means learning all over again and giving up your routine. Thirty years ago, when parents in the West were excluded from the care given to their sick newborn babies, the idea that prevailed was that you must protect these delicate babies from any risk of outside infection. The mothers and fathers had to accept this transfer of responsibility to medical and paramedical staff. The doctor became, at this time, a sort of intermediary between the parents and their baby; he could see and touch their baby; they had to be content with seeing it from a distance, without understanding all the tubes and machinery it was surrounded by; they suffered at not being able to do anything, they suffered in silence. That period is happily on its way out; gradually the significance of the initial mother-baby bond is regaining all its importance, and the parents' role from the very first days of life is again given its proper value. Born too soon (and increasingly more so moreover) or sick at birth, these fragile babies need non-stressful surroundings where the mother has a place, and a place in the foreground. The value of the power of a reassuring voice, of a familiar scent, of gentle loving contact is increased when it is a tiny baby who is dumbly suffering; we are aware of the trauma caused by permanent lighting, incessant background noise, a lack of respect for sleep, the pain of a blood test . . .

Today, it is an established fact that a baby grows when it is well; then, its need for oxygen decreases and it emerges from the critical period more rapidly. Our mission as carers is to find a balance between what is of necessity disagreeable but imperative and what we can do to soften the traumatising effect of some of our actions; and it is there that the kangaroo mother technique comes into its own, particularly in developed countries, notably because work can be done with the family's collaboration. The kangaroo mother technique is also a complementary method of care that is entirely special. Every year, new neonatal care units are adopting it and introducing it into their practice, first for an hour, then for more. When these units are designed in years to come they should take into account the need for a place for kangaroo mothers.

For more than ten years, the Swedes have been interested in the kangaroo mother method. Its application has almost become a routine there. If the mother and baby can't be sent home, then the home must come to the hospital and flats have been organised so that parents can live there with their tiny baby until a reasonable time for discharge. The incubator is installed in the flat and a thick cover is placed over it to replicate the all-important alternation of night and day. All the techniques that can benefit mothers and children are adopted in northern countries, the kangaroo technique as well as NIDCAP (Newborn Individualized Developmental Care and Assessment Program).

In the UK, where as many as 80,000 babies a year need special care, neonatal units are also beginning to use the kangaroo method, but one of the great obstacles remains their lack of space: all too often the units are too small, and it is impossible even to put a chair and a mother there for more than a few hours every day. What has become known as 'kangaroo care' – skin-to-skin contact for short periods – is widely practised in these units. A recent article in the *British Medical Journal* by Professor Neil Marlow of Queens Medical Centre, Nottingham, points out that in western settings kangaroo care has a three-fold purpose: 'improved contact between mother and infant (and father and infant), quicker establishment of breastfeeding, and a shorter stay in hospital'. However he goes on to say that 'In my experience it is not universally welcomed by all mothers.' This he puts down to 'embarrassment' in the 'busy, hard-pressed and often impersonal environment' of the neonatal unit, and his article criticises the 'rigid systematic programme of care' that is currently prevalent. He concludes that kangaroo mother care forms 'a valuable and evidence-based part in the repertory of increasingly baby-sensitive care'. A UK charity, Bliss (www.bliss.org.uk), has been established to help families with premature babies, and they recommend kangaroo care, but only if the baby is well enough. They advise talking to the staff at the unit

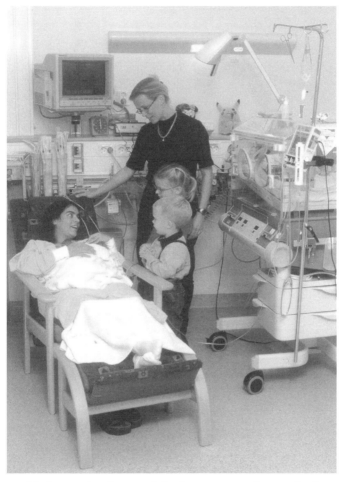

Modern technology and the kangaroo mother method
make good partners

first and finding a quiet, comfortable place to sit, when 'you may be able to cuddle for twenty minutes or so. Different babies can cope with varying lengths of cuddles – when ready you may go on for hours!' One father of a very premature baby (born after only 25 weeks and 4 days of gestation, and a month later weighing only 1,000g) describes on the Internet his joy when his tiny boy reached his first birthday. In his diary of those perilous weeks after his son Archie's birth, he records on the sixteenth day: 'Sarah and I had a kangaroo hold tonight. Skin to skin . . . Lovely!'

Belgium has also followed the trend and a superb neonatal care unit, with top technology and humanised methods will soon open in Brussels.

France remains somewhat timid, but not for much longer, one hopes. Historically, one of the first kangaroo units in France was that at the hospital of Antoine-Béclère. There, when the baby needs to stay in hospital for several days, the incubator is put in the room and the mother can stay with her baby day and night and carry it for some of the time if she so wishes; though carrying the baby and breastfeeding it are not made a priority. Another kangaroo unit which is particularly interesting is that at the Central hospital at Créteil, created by Dr Christiane Huraux and her team, and since taken over by Dr Anne Cortey. At Créteil, it is not just a question of the incubator being placed in the mother's room, the mother undertakes to live at the hospital for as long as the baby does, and she is encouraged to breastfeed and carry her baby for as long as she can. The different techniques of feeding milk to the

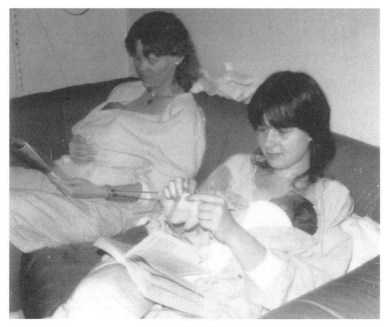

Some read and knit . . .

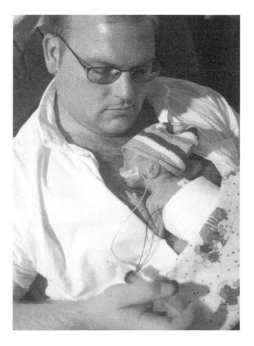

Others give the baby its feed . . .

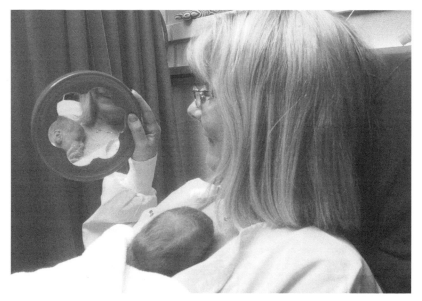

One can read this western mother's joy in the
mirror she is holding . . .

baby are taught here and everything is done to help the mother in the arduous task of giving a premature baby milk. Although few in number the unit's paediatric nurses are trained to respect the strength of the initial mother-baby bond and to feel that they are participating in an adventure of humanising neonatal care. Of course, they know that it is more work for them, but they accept it because they can measure the benefits of direct skin-to-skin contact: which not only promotes the mother and baby's wellbeing, a better mutual understanding and communication between the two, but stimulates the baby's growth and lessens the pain after a blood test or injection. With the backing of carers, some mothers have even gone so far as carrying their baby for the full twenty-four hours a day, like real Colombian mothers. Breast milk, too often neglected and mistrusted in favour of commercial products that are easier to administer, is favoured, because the kangaroo mother method encourages successful breastfeeding. As soon as they are thirty-two weeks old, if their state is not critical, the babies are welcomed into the unit that, despite numerous demands, works not only for the mothers but also for the professionals who like coming to see what is going on or be initiated by the team working there.

In Brest, where the kangaroo mother method and NIDCAP have dynamically coexisted for a number of years, in Strasbourg, Marseilles, Nantes, Lorient, Valenciennes and many other French towns, similar initiatives are on the increase. For the moment, there is no co-ordination of groups that would allow all the teams dedicated to improving the care given to fragile babies to communicate, have meetings, exchange experiences or compare their results. If there were such an organisation, it would dismiss the doubts of those who are tempted by the experience but are still hesitating.

Nevertheless the situation is getting better. A French association for Kangaroo Mothers was formed several years ago (prev@club-internet.fr) under the benevolent presidency of a paediatrician, Véronique Prévost, and will shortly publish a French directory of the different centres that favour a more humanised approach to neonatalogy, and primarily the kangaroo mother method.

France, with its own special rhythm, is advancing slowly but steadily in the direction of change. Carrying the baby in the kangaroo position, even if it is just for a few hours a day, will gradually become the order of the day in French maternity units. Using breast milk for the premature baby will come next, once the difficulties of its practice and the training necessary to guarantee its success have been recognised. Early discharge from hospital and the participation of the parents night and day, on the other hand, will probably be more difficult to adopt, among families as well as professionals. But, there too, it is a question of time and kangaroo babies are without doubt going to become more and more numerous in France in the future.

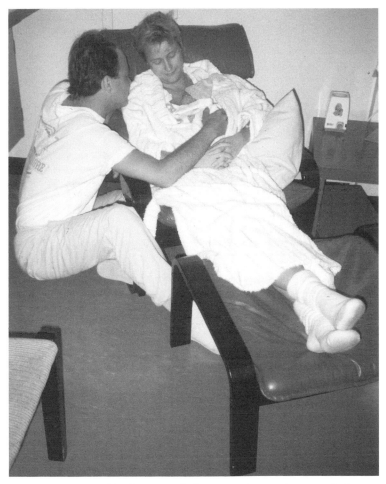

What more could a kangaroo baby want than to be snuggled up
against its mother, with its daddy not far away . . .?

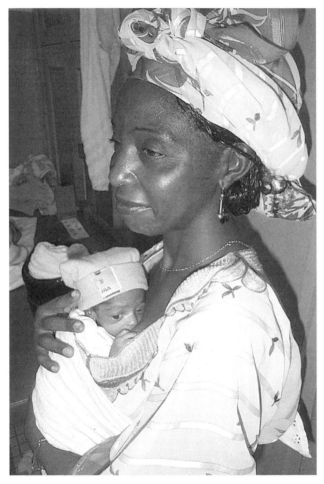

There is such pride on the face of this African
kangaroo mother

6

Growing Support in Africa

The newborn baby unit at La Quintinie hospital, Douala, Cameroon

Some years ago, a team at Douala, made up of Béatrice, a paediatrician, and Anne, a nurse, came to Bogotá to learn the kangaroo mother method. On their return to Cameroon, the head of the unit, Dr Odette Guifo, a dynamic paediatrician, supervised the setting up of the kangaroo mother programme. It was no easy job. Douala, one of Cameroon's big cities, has a very hot, humid climate, and in the beginning kangaroo mothers found the method much too sweaty and exhausting. It needed a great deal of persuasion to convince them to carry their baby all the time, but they set to it and set to it well, and very soon this unit will begin forming other national centres.

In the hospital at Douala, the newborn baby unit is equipped with incubators and cots, but has no ventilation or air-conditioning, which makes work difficult. The incubators are full of minute, adorable shrimps, which is impressive. Dr Guifo has developed a system of feeding by tube every thirty minutes, and carried out by the mothers themselves and a big clock has been put up on the wall to remind them when it is time. The organisation is impressive. Seated beside the incubators, some of the mothers carry their baby kangaroo-style, held in a band of green phosphorescent synthetic Lycra bought in the local market. There are rows of babies of 1,000 g, 1,200 g and 1,300 g. As a general rule the mothers are clumsy and give little support to their tiny baby's neck. As soon as the baby is capable of accepting half its ration using a tube, suckling the baby at the breast can begin. Grandmothers are also there to help carry the baby and listen attentively to all the advice.

Justine and her friends

Justine is proud of the fact that she has given birth to a pair of twins and both have survived. She spends her days at the hospital waiting impatiently for the moment when her two daughters will be with her in the kangaroo mother and baby unit which is separated by a simple partition from the neonatal care unit. She knows that she must wait until she is able to breast-feed before Dr Béatrice will agree to hand them over to her. So she spends her morning expressing her milk, feeding it to her little girls, then carrying them in the kangaroo position alternately. Sometimes her mother comes to help her. The stools in the hospital are very uncomfortable and she would really love to be in bed with her baby girls.

To her right is Alice, the grandmother of little Anita.

Anita's mother died giving birth. She was HIV positive, but happily it seems that Anita has escaped this. At the beginning Alice did not want to carry her granddaughter, partly through grief after her daughter's death and also because she thought that the baby would not survive. But since she has been carrying her in the kangaroo position, her attitude has changed: she has become attached to this tiny scrap of a thing which is all that remains to her of her own child.

To Justine's left is a pair of twins, Jacques and Cédric, carried by their aunts Cindy and Collette, Amande's two sisters. Amande underwent a caesarean four days ago and is still too weak to get up. It needed all Dr Guifo's powers of persuasion to convince her to come to the unit to give breast milk to her two boys.

The department is jam-packed and very rapidly the mothers pass to the kangaroo mother-baby unit. The mothers begin to get enthused by this method. The oldest have understood the programme perfectly and have discovered that, even in a climate so hot and humid as this, their tiny baby is going to lose weight and have frozen hands if they do not carry it all the time in the kangaroo position. They learn to recruit a member of their family to help them bathe the baby and wash nappies or walk for a little while in the hospital to relax. The person in the family who helps them also learns the kangaroo method in this way. It is only when the mothers feel capable of doing all these things at home that the baby's discharge from hospital is authorised.

Thanks to the kangaroo mother method, the mother

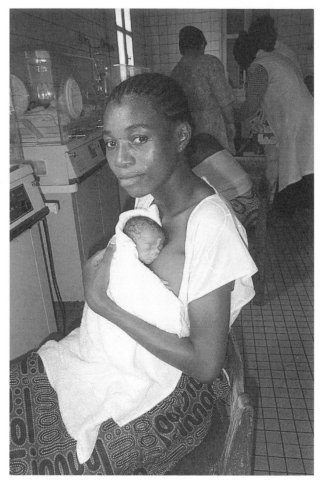

Justine, mother of the tiny twins

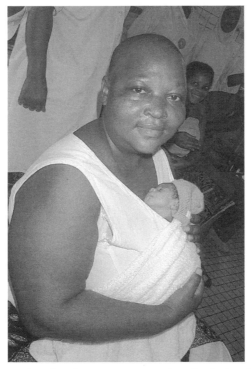

Alice is a grandmother kangaroo. Every day she feels a little more love for her orphaned granddaughter Anita. She knows that she will take proper care of her

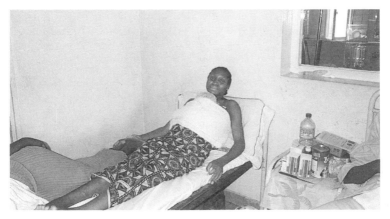

The kangaroo mother-baby beds are very uncomfortable and make carrying the baby for twenty-four hours a day difficult. But all that is needed to make life easier are a few large cushions with washable loose covers . . .

and baby's stay in hospital is shorter and that pleases everybody. The babies have fewer infections and return more quickly to their family; the incubators are freed up more rapidly and the number of hospitalised babies in the department can be almost doubled. Needless to say, the staff need to be organised so that they are not snowed under, but the mothers participate actively in the caring.

The outpatient clinic

When the clinic first started, so Dr Béatrice told me, the mothers would come back with their baby wrapped in a piece of cloth, because they found carrying their baby inside their clothes generally impractical. Cameroon women are quite coquettish and their clothes are tailored to mould their body. Then they discovered that their baby grew more quickly if they carried it next to the skin, and now they come to the consultation with their baby in the kangaroo position. Let us hope that that will continue.

The situation in other African countries

While everything is going well in Cameroon, kangaroo mother care is rapidly taking root in other African countries, with South Africa leading the way. The country has embarked upon an ambitious programme to spread the kangaroo method throughout its territories. Kenya, Malawi and Uganda have also started to develop this

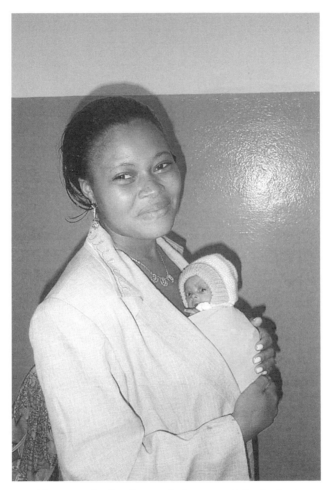

The consultation is a real pleasure – it looks just
like a fashion show

method in their capitals, while Ethiopia has had the kangaroo programme in place more or less for five years. Togo and, somewhat tentatively, Senegal and Nigeria have also undertaken it. Finally that island which is so beautiful and so destitute – Madagascar – also uses kangaroo mother care in the huge maternity hospital at Antananarivo – Befalatanana maternity hospital. So what do Madagascan mothers think?

The kangaroo mother programme in Madagascar

Yvonne and Aimée have had responsibility for the kangaroo programme for several years, and last year in collaboration with the Madagascan Ministry of Health and with Unicef's support they embarked upon an ambitious project to spread the kangaroo mother method.

Antananarivo is a pretty town, coated in grey dust and with innumerable steps. Beside the willows there are very beautiful trees loaded with lilac-coloured flowers: these are jacarandas, a real treat for the eyes. Befalatanana maternity hospital, where my colleagues work, has a newborn baby unit equipped with eight incubators and thirty cradles hanging like hammocks; there are 12,000 births a year there. It is a big, well ventilated hospital; the staff are helpful and that is important: the Madagascans are very likeable, courteous people.

Kangaroo training at Befalatanana maternity hospital

The mothers sit on hard wooden benches. Like mothers the world over they are ready to do anything to save their tiny babies, including spending twelve hours sitting on these uncomfortable seats. The room set aside for kangaroo training is next to the neonatal department; it is jam-packed. Véronique is there with her tiny baby daughter weighing 1,200 g; Rindra with Olivier, her minute 1,000 g shrimp; Jeanne with Terry, her baby son of 1,500 g, who is very lazy about sucking; there is also Cédric, 1,300 g, the tiny baby belonging to Tica, a kangaroo mother who has emerged as a 'leader'.

All these tiny premature babies still have to be fed by tube to receive their nourishment, for they are not yet able to suck their mother's breast efficiently. The mothers have learned to express their milk and under Yvonne and Aimée's directions look after the feeding by tube themselves: this lessens the carers' workload in the unit, as there are too few of them.

One of the fundamental points at Befalatanana has been teaching the mothers the different techniques of feeding and gavage. You have to recognise that nature has done things well: breast milk for a premature baby is in fact different from the milk mothers produce for a baby that has gone full term; it contains more salt and more proteins and so satisfies the special requirements of a premature baby. Whether one is in a developing country or a developed one, when it is possible to feed a baby with its mother's breast milk, it has a better chance of quality survival.

Promoting breast milk

These Madagascan mothers spend the whole morning and the whole afternoon in the kangaroo training room and only leave for lunch; they express their milk themselves and give it warm and clean to their baby through a tube. They have learned to measure the residues which remain their baby's stomach before introducing the tube. Weight is measured daily, and they are greatly encouraged when they see their baby growing and beginning to suck direct from the breast, for then they know that they will soon be able to leave the hospital. Every mother in every culture does not really feel herself to be a 'true' mother until the day she can go home with her little baby.

Tica is proud of herself, so is her husband. He has been given permission to enter the training room and he takes great pleasure in carrying his baby. As a result he will come back almost every day to re-experience this pleasure. Some of the grandparents are there too. The room is very, very hot . . . And, on this particular day, there is nothing that can be done to alleviate the sluggish atmosphere. A baby has died in the department; it weighed only 700 g and could not survive. Its mother carried it for the two days it survived next to her skin; the fact that she took part in caring for her baby will help her to cope better in the grieving process, but it is still hard all the same . . . Rindra is attending to her baby's every need – Olivier weighs only 1,000 g and she has decided, and is proclaiming it loud and strong, that her tiny son is going to live. In fact, several weeks later, Olivier was able to leave the maternity hospital with his mother now an expert in the kangaroo method. She pulled him through, well and truly.

The kangaroo room has always been full ever since it was created and new mothers join the old ones who kindly show them the ropes in this great kangaroo mothers' adventure at Antananarivo, while Yvonne and Aimée are always there, attentive and ready to help and accompany them.

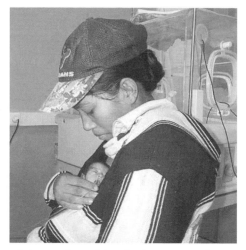

This mother is intensely sad for she knows that her baby will not live, but she finds comfort in being able to help him a little

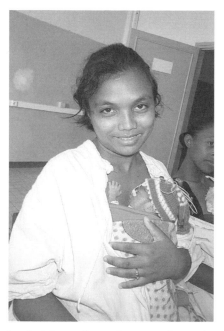

Tica will be a 'leader' throughout the several months that her baby will be in hospital. It is very important to have some well trained mothers for they can offer psychological support to the ever-anxious new arrivals

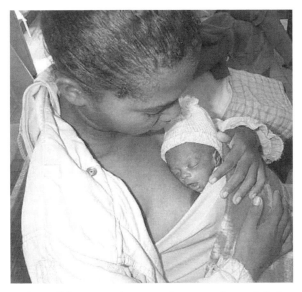

Rindra still has some long weeks to get through before
she can think of taking her baby home

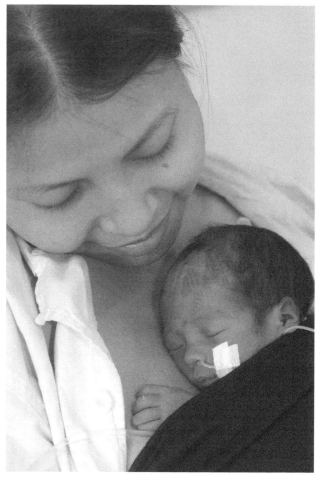

How secure this little baby feels nestled
against his mother's skin

7

Thousands of Babies Saved in India and the Far East

Kangaroo mother care in Vietnam

For more than ten years, the kangaroo mother method has been practised at the hospital of Uong Bi, north of Hanoi, under the direction of a young paediatrician, Dr Nga Nguyen. After reading some articles on the method, Dr Nga went to Bogotá to observe the method being applied, and then set up a very pretty Kangaroo Mother programme at her hospital, in a little house in the hospital gardens. The paediatric department has very few incubators and the mothers are generally used as 'human incubators' from the moment their premature baby is born. Once the baby is stabilised, it is transferred with its mother into this little house until it has grown sufficiently and can be discharged.

The north of Hanoi is a region where numerous ethnic minorities live, often in villages a long way from the town; this is why families have to stay at the hospital and wait until their baby has gained enough weight for them to have a check-up only once a week and not every day. If they left too early, it would be impossible for the family to come back every day as it should. The kangaroo rules in

Vietnam are now well established and Dr Nga as well as all the staff in the paediatric department are very proud, and justly so, of the work they have achieved.

For the last two years, along with another flagship programme in the country, that of Ho Chi Minh city, an ambitious campaign has begun to spread the use of the kangaroo mother method, with the assistance of APPEL, a French NGO. More than twenty regional centres are currently being formed or have been formed already in the two former centres. Dr Nga sometimes complains about the slowness with which the new centres are launching their programme: she knows that, probably, she ought to go and give them a helping hand.

The application of the kangaroo mother method in Ho Chi Minh-City, the capital of the country, is co-ordinated by Dr Luong Kim Chi; it is taking place in the largest public maternity hospital in the city, the Tu Du Hospital, whose neonatal department is always overstretched. This maternity hospital deals with 30,000 births every year, an astronomical figure if one considers the average number of births in a French maternity hospital, which is around 2,500 a year. So the kangaroo mother method has provided an appreciable solution to limit the occupation of the incubators. The tiny premature babies who still are unable to suck efficiently do not stay on in the neonatal department but are transferred to a large room right next to it. Here, under the supervision of a kangaroo nurse, their mothers are taught to express their milk and to feed the babies by tube themselves. When it is deemed that the baby is gaining sufficient weight, it will go home with the

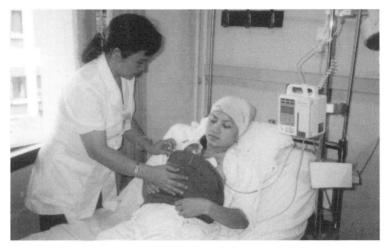

As soon as the baby is born, it is stabilised by nestling it skin to skin against its mother, who thus takes the place of the incubator

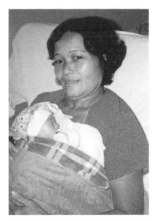

When the climate is very hot and humid as it is in Ho Chi Minh City, a cloth towel is placed between the baby's cheek and the mother's skin to prevent sweating

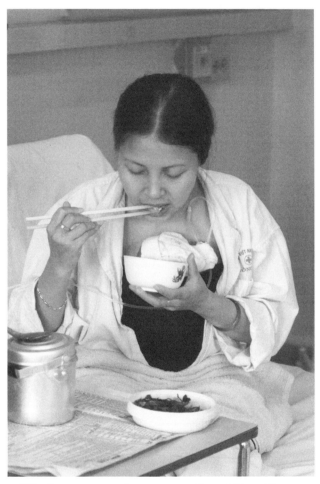

Whether you are a kangaroo mother at Uong Bi or a
kangaroo mother in Bogotá . . . it's the same story
except for a few small details

feeding tube and return regularly to the outpatient clinic, which is well organised but always full to overflowing, for check-ups. The biggest problem for Dr Nga and Dr Chi is undoubtedly being overwhelmed with work; they have had the know-how to develop and spread the kangaroo mother method in Vietnam but their work is far from being finished.

The situation in India

In India the kangaroo method appeared several years ago as the only efficient technique to cut down the death rate and improve the nutrition of babies who had a low birth weight. The debate now centres on an urgent need to agree whether to create centres of excellence or to spread the kangaroo mother method in the villages. Bearing in mind the fact that in the Indian mega-cities, more than 60 per cent of births take place in hospital, it seems to me that creating kangaroo mother method centres of excellence in the big university centres is of prime importance if the method is to be accepted, and that the second stage should be spreading the kangaroo mother method to less sophisticated hospitals and to local care centres in order to create a coherent network for supervising babies that are born with a low birth weight.

For several years now, many teams from the big Indian university hospitals, made up of a paediatric department head and a nurse, have come to Colombia to observe the kangaroo programme, and five kangaroo mother method centres of excellence have been set up between 2003 and 2004 in Chennai (Madras), Lucknow, New Delhi, Chandigarh and finally in Mumbai (Bombay). The idea is that these centres will become centres of reference and training for all the hospitals and dispensaries that wish to be initiated into the method. It is still too soon to make an assessment, but everything leads one to believe that the kangaroo mother method will save numerous lives of babies born preterm or of low birth weight on the Indian continent.

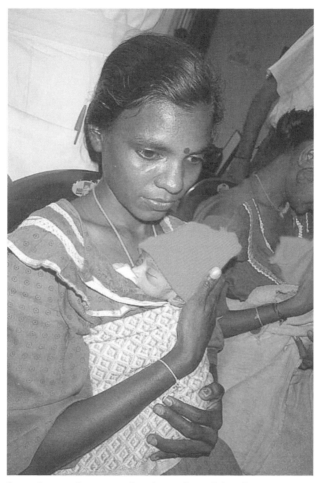

Too often, the mothers' comfort is neglected, but how can one ask a woman to carry her baby night and day, when she has only the metal bars of her bed to rest her back?

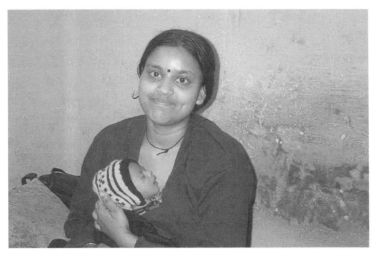

Saroj has had twins and for the last fifteen days she has carried them in the kangaroo position at home with the help of her mother-in-law. She is very proud of her and of her family

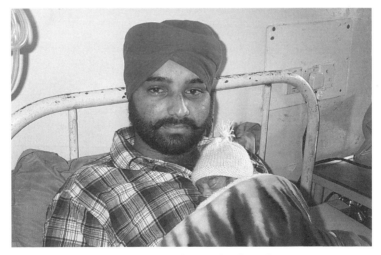

Father and mother share the work when there are twins

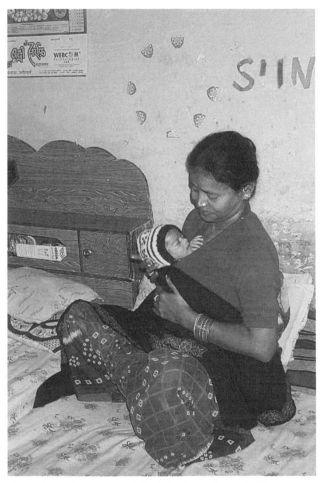

One of Saroj's twins now weighs 1,900g and would like to get out of the kangaroo position. Many babies in India are undernourished and ask to come out of the kangaroo position at a weight lower than Colombian babies. With this lower weight, these Indian babies are already mature enough to regulate their own temperature

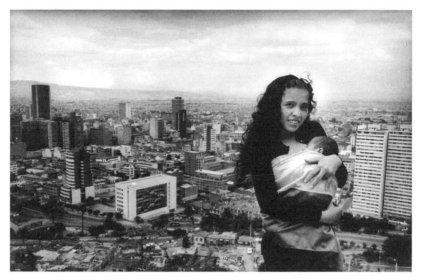

A spectacular view of Bogotá, birthplace of the
kangaroo mother method

Conclusion

Let us hear what a final witness, another kangaroo mother, has to say :

Despite the crying need for intimacy and comfort, and all those moments when the 'kangaroo' was being interrupted to administer a drip or a feeding tube, the times spent together were unbelievably intense. The exchanges between my baby and me were so strong that we were as one, just as when he was still in my womb. It was as though we were on a journey together, escaping through windows, leapfrogging clouds to discover the freedom that was so cruelly lacking for us. If I could have . . . I would have remained all day and all night with my baby against me. But with my caesarean I couldn't endure more than an hour of sitting on that chair, and in any case that was the rule they set down. After an hour, they took away my baby to put back his sensors and return him to the incubator . . .

From experience I know that all, or almost all, parents the world over need to feel close to their baby, that they are capable of participating in the caring their baby receives at birth, and that they have the skills for it. They are the ones who are the most faithful adherents of the kangaroo method; they are the ones who end up bringing about the changes necessary in today's neonatal care units. In writing this book, my wish has been to arm them with the correct information, so that they can make moves in this direction and follow their heart.

At the risk of repeating myself, I say again that kangaroo mother care is not meant to be a substitute for the methods of caring that are normally employed in big modern, well equipped maternity hospitals in the West, that are unstinting towards the newborn. But it is for all fragile, delicate babies a precious adjunct that will help them fare better and develop better. Even tiny babies who do not present any special problem can profit from the benefits of this method, which is for all parents the world over a marvellous way of getting to know their child and of learning very quickly to take care of this little being who has so much need of them. What is good for the countries of the South is also good for those of the North, and in light of the knowledge at our disposal today, it is more than time, it seems to me, to introduce this method in a systematic way into every neonatal care unit in the rich, so-called developed countries.

Conversely, obviously, I also hope that, in the near future, the sophisticated technical methods available in the North will also be available in the South and that all the babies in the world, without distinction of race, will be able to profit from them. In the meantime, the kangaroo method is there and helps us save thousands of lives every year. It is certainly not enough, but it is already considerable.

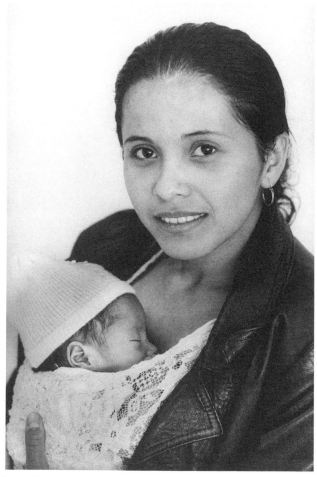

This Colombian mother shows such confidence in the future,
as does her little one who is sleeping so peacefully

Further Information

The Kangaroo Foundation

The Kangaroo Foundation was created ten years ago by health professionals who wanted to give neonatalogy a human face. Its aim is to spread the kangaroo mother method in good conditions, and promote breastfeeding at the same time. The Kangaroo Foundation is also researching possible improvements in the kangaroo method, as a result of the follow-ups and evaluations of different kangaroo mother programmes set up throughout the world. For than forty-four teams from twenty-five countries, principally developing ones, have come to Colombia to observe and train in this method. These initiatives, that have already been taken, or are currently underway, correspond to a real need for better knowledge of appropriate care for preterm babies or babies that have a low birth weight in developing countries. This includes the application of the kangaroo mother method, but also other aspects of care given to fragile babies: nutrition, detection and treatment of eventual after-effects, quality of the mother-baby relationship, outpatient follow-up, etc. The Kangaroo Foundation is not short of imagination or competent professionals to continue its mission of spreading the method and evaluating it – missions which have become even more important than the kangaroo rules set out by the World Health Organisation which were published in 2003. The main obstacle to action by our foundation is lack of funding. In the world in which we are living, it is difficult to encounter nongovernmental organisations that are interested in supporting long-term, sustained activities; in general they are more interested in immediate and tangible results, and do not wish to invest in scientific research in developing countries. They consider this claim superfluous. In fact, an analysis of the studies carried out on the kangaroo mother method shows that most of the work done is carried out in rich countries, that is to say, in the place where only 10 per cent of babies that have a low birth weight could profit by it. For this reason we must address our warm thanks to the Swiss NGO which has supported us for the last ten years: the World Laboratory La Fondation Kangourou is working not only in Colombia now but in different kangaroo centres established around the world. For several years, it has undertaken to create a kangaroo network through the Internet: http://kangaroo.javeriana.edu.co. Registration is free and health professionals who would like to create their own kangaroo mother method centre can access on this site the kangaroo mother method application rules and the list of scientific publications relating to developed and developing countries. You will also find resumés of work presented at meetings of INK (International Network of the Kangaroo Mother Method) since 1996. The page is more complete in English than in Spanish and needs to be translated into other languages, but voluntary help is limited . . .

Fundación Canguro
Carrera 7,No. 46-20, Apta 2001
Bogotá,Colombia

Some Recommendations for Health Professionals

Here are fifteen essential rules to promote the development, application and spread of kangaroo mother care in your institution.

1. You should be aware that the kangaroo mother method must have multidisciplinary skills: for this reason it is better to begin setting up kangaroo mother care with a team made up of, as a minimum, a paediatrician and a nurse who are already aware of the method. To this should then be added: a psychologist, a nutritionist, a social worker and a physiotherapist etc.

2. You should be personally persuaded that the kangaroo mother method is a bonus in the practice of neonatalogy, and that the families of the babies hospitalised in the unit are capable of learning what they need to know in order to look after their baby, without risk and efficiently.

3. You should participate in or be present at the application of kangaroo mother care in a unit which has the same characteristics as yours.

4. You should make the most comprehensive collection of documentation on the kangaroo mother method, including audiovisual material, scientific studies, and protocols applied in other units or in other countries.

5. You should distribute this documentation to all the staff in your unit, then organise a meeting for general information – to which you should invite a representative of the hospital administration – and describe in a practical way the kangaroo mother method to all the participants present.

6. You should begin the kangaroo mother method with mothers in the unit who would like to use it.

7. You should begin the kangaroo mother method, once you have the agreement of both parents, with the most stable babies who will not pose problems. The baby can be 'monitored' from the beginning (oxygenation, heart rate) to reinforce the confidence of the carers and parents.

8. You should evaluate and adapt, if need be, the kangaroo rules that can be applied in the department; you should publish them in a written form.

9. You should register and follow up the results with a base of kangaroo data, first of all up to forty weeks after conception (the length of a normal pregnancy and point zero for each baby), then for at least a year following. It is the only way to be able to compare your own results (mortality, morbidity rate, length of hospitalisation, costs, length of breastfeeding, after-effects, etc.) with those obtained from other units, but also to be able to respond to eventual external criticisms that the introduction of kangaroo mother care, like any other change of practice, may give rise to.

10. You should not forget to ask the families to give evidence: the kangaroo families are always ready to co-operate, it is one of their special things. They feel strongly and are confident that they are right – after all, they are the ones who do the work and pull these tiny fragile babies through.

11. You should try to obtain the approval of the Minister of Health and get the kangaroo mother method

included on the list of official medical and paramedical training.

12. You should look to transform your unit into a pilot centre for training in kangaroo mother care and present the results obtained at national and international congresses.

13. You should be ready to teach at other hospitals where the experience acquired in the kangaroo mother method will spread to health professionals: they in their turn would welcome being initiated rapidly.

14. You should broadcast the kangaroo mother method on TV, radio, in the newspapers: the media are interested in the kangaroo mother method; you must satisfy their demands.

15. You should identify and adapt the best kangaroo practice to the level of development of the institution concerned by participating in national and international workshops on kangaroo mother care. Every two years an international congress takes place, in which not only the problems of spreading the kangaroo mother method are analysed, but also the different methods of possible adaptation which vary according to the centre concerned – kangaroo mother care may vary according to whether it is being used in a rural hospital in Africa or a Brazilian hospital. The World Health Organisation takes part in this congress and their booklet published in 2003 is an outcome of these congresses.